Sex, Technology and Public Health

Mark Davis
Monash University, Australia

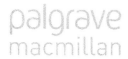

palgrave
macmillan

First published 2009 by
PALGRAVE MACMILLAN

Palgrave Macmillan in the UK is an imprint of Macmillan Publishers Limited,
registered in England, company number 785998, of Houndmills, Basingstoke,
Hampshire RG21 6XS.

Palgrave Macmillan in the US is a division of St Martin's Press LLC,
175 Fifth Avenue, New York, NY 10010.

Palgrave Macmillan is the global academic imprint of the above companies
and has companies and representatives throughout the world.

Palgrave® and Macmillan® are registered trademarks in the United States,
the United Kingdom, Europe and other countries.

ISBN-13: 978-0-230-52562-7   hardback
ISBN-10: 0-230-52562-8   hardback

This book is printed on paper suitable for recycling and made from fully
managed and sustained forest sources. Logging, pulping and manufacturing
processes are expected to conform to the environmental regulations of the
country of origin.

A catalogue record for this book is available from the British Library.

Library of Congress Cataloging-in-Publication Data

Davis, Mark (Mark David McGregor)
   Sex, technology, and public health / Mark Davis.
       p. ; cm.
   Includes bibliographical references and index.
   ISBN-13: 978-0-230-52562-7 (hardback : alk. paper)
   ISBN-10: 0-230-52562-8 (hardback : alk. paper)
       1. Hygiene, Sexual. 2. Public health. 3. Communication and
   technology. 4. Communication and sex. 5. Internet. I. Title.
   [DNLM: 1. Public Health–trends. 2. Sexual Behavior. 3. Internet.
   4. Sexually Transmitted Diseases. 5. Technology. WA 100 D263s 2009]
   RA788.D38 2009
   613–dc22   2008029923

10   9   8   7   6   5   4   3   2   1
18 17 16 15 14 13 12 11 10 09

Transferred to Digital Printing in 2014

Contents

Acknowledgements   vii

1   Introduction   1
    The rise of the technosexuals   2
    Sexuality, technology and public health   6
    Defining public health   11
    Technosexual citizenship?   15
    Overview   18

2   Technologies and Sexual Citizenship   22
    Questing avatars   25
    Viagra cyborgs   32
    Technosexual citizenship as relational ethics   38

3   Internet-Mediated Sexual Practices   48
    E-dating as a sexual health risk   49
    Techno-determinism and cyber-perversity   51
    E-dating as reflexive practice   58
    Narcissism and other challenges   66

4   HIV Bio-Technologies and Sexual Practice   75
    The advent of effective HIV treatment   77
    The treatment optimism narrative   81
    Reflexive HIV treatment   85
    Hyper-technologisation and sexual cultures   91

5   Innovation and Imperative   98
    Gift and contagion   101
    Altruism   108
    Risk and its forensic turning   112

6   Technological Visibilities   122
    Technology and visibility   125
    Spectacular risk, ethnographic media and forensic research   128
    The politics of technosexual transgressions   134

7 The Reshaping of Public Health   143
   Authority and public health   145
   Medicalisation and de-medicalisation   148
   Democratic health care?   153
   Dialogical public health   156

8 Conclusion   163
   Self-animation   164
   Governing through danger/cure   167
   The passing of 'public' health   170

Bibliography   173

Index   189

Acknowledgements

For their advice and support, I wish to thank Professor Paul Flowers, Glasgow Caledonian University, Professor Corinne Squire, University of East London, and Dr Suzanne Fraser, Monash University. For their helpful advice, I would like to thank the anonymous reviewers and editors at Palgrave Macmillan. I also want to thank Dr Peter Hengstberger and Brent Jones for making space for me in their home in South East Queensland so I could complete the manuscript.

I have used quotations in this book from interviews published in articles I wrote for several research projects:

Transitions in HIV Management: The Role of Innovative Health Technologies, UK Economic and Social Research and Medical Research Councils, Innovative Health Technologies Programme (Grant: L218252011), Paul Flowers (Principal Investigator), Graham Hart (Investigator), John Imrie (Investigator), Mark Davis (Investigator), Marsha Rosengarten (Researcher), Jamie Frankis (Researcher).

Sexual risk behaviour and relation to anti-retroviral therapy in HIV positive gay men, UK Medical Research Council (Grant: G98116 43) Judith Stephenson (Principal Investigator), John Imrie (Principal Investigator), Graham Hart (Investigator), Oliver Davidson (Investigator), Ian Williams (Investigator)

The Internet and HIV, UK Medical Research Council (Grant: GO 100159). I am grateful for my colleagues in those projects for their support and assistance. Jonathan Elford (Principal Investigator), Lorraine Sherr (Investigator), Graham Hart, (Investigator) Graham Bolding (Researcher).

I would like to extend my thanks to my colleagues in these research projects. I am particularly grateful for the men and women who agreed to be interviewed for these research projects.

1
Introduction

Sex and technology have connections that are taken for granted and surprising. Many of us have become accustomed to dealing with spam email promoting products such as Viagra. Much of this email traffic is unseen as our email servers channel it away from our inboxes. But occasionally something slips through to remind us of the seemingly enormous and definitely relentless sexual potential of the internet. Late night television carries advertisements for e-dating websites and mobile phone based pornography, suggesting the existence of a niche market of sexually-interested insomniacs. After drugs such as Viagra and the internet, it is possible to regard the connections between sex and technology as obvious and perhaps everyday. But it is worth reflecting on how it is to live with sexual practices that are sustained, extended and reconfigured through various bio- and communication technologies. The new forms of sexuopharmacy, such as Viagra, have become extremely profitable (Tiefer, 2006). These products are said to be altering how the sexual body, experience, and pleasure are understood. *Match.com* (accessed 10 August 2008), an e-dating website catering to opposite and same sex attracted men and women, is said to claim nine million subscribers (Arvidsson, 2006). Online dating services designed so that people can meet in the flesh, social networking sites, and other forms of interactive media have given rise to new possibilities for intimacy and sexual relating, imagined and materialised. It is also important to recognise that such bio- and communication technologies further each other. For example, the internet-based self-prescribing of Viagra suggests how bio-technologies can be extended through the internet, but also how the internet finds value in its capacity to make such bio-technologies available. For instance, *Viagra.com* helps citizens in general decide if they need a prescription.

It is also the case that connections between sex and technology have come into view as both problems and solutions for public health. For example, there are concerns that the transmission of sexually transmitted infections, including HIV, is linked with Viagra and the internet. Practitioners are using the internet to extend interventions concerning sexually transmitted infections, HIV, and related concerns. Some are calling for an approach that would seek to govern the relationship between sex and technology in accord with public health rationalities of disease control. It seems that new forms of public health governance are coming into being because of the connections between sex and technology. It remains an open question whether these efforts will be effective. Some of them may even be counterproductive. Public health is imposing itself on the sexual uses of technology, but there is reason to explore how public health is itself changing in technologically-mediated societies. It is crucial to consider these developments in terms of the assumptions they make concerning social action, and the effects they may have in our sexual and intimate lives.

This book addresses the links between sexual practice, bio- and communication technologies, and public health, with reference to sexually transmitted infections and HIV. I will adopt two main strategies. Part of this book will develop a social science account of the links between sex, technology and public health. On that basis, this book will also consider how public health is addressing the connections between sex and technology.

The sections to follow establish the conceptual frame for this book and outline its structure. In the first section, I will introduce the notion of 'technosexuality' as a way of drawing together the different kinds of connections that are being produced between sex and technology. In the next sections, I outline the key public health interests in this new mixing of technologies and sexual practices, and establish how public health governance will be defined in this book. As a way of situating the argument, I will then provide an overview of research that can help illuminate the relationships between sex, technology and public health governance. In the final section of this chapter, I briefly outline the argument of this book and provide an overview of the chapters to follow.

The rise of the technosexuals

The connection between technology and sexuality has been with us for some time, particularly with regard to the internet. In his account of the information society, Manuel Castells made reference to the 1980s French *Minitel* computer network, noting how its economic viability was due in part to its popularity as a method of dating (2000). It seems that almost as soon as the internet came into use, its sexual potential was put to work. It appears that the sexual uses of the internet and related technologies are now understood by some to comprise 'techno-sexuality' and to have many implications for intimate life and civil society. I want to suggest that this notion of technosexuality can be extended to include bio-technology such as Viagra, and its association with communication technologies.

Technosexuality would seem to be an obvious, fairly transparent neologism for a book such as this. But the term has an interesting, if short, history. Ken Plummer used the term "techno-sex" as a way of characterising telephone sex and to make the point that such sexual uses of communication technology had specific value as safe sex for societies living after HIV and AIDS (1995: 136). Gordo-Lopez and Cleminson used the term 'technosexual' in their book which used Foucauldian ideas to address sexuality and technology in general (Gordo-Lopez & Cleminson, 2004). But the term technosexual appears to have significance outside academia. Calvin Klein Corporation and some other commercial organisations have attempted to trademark 'technosexual' in the United States. Calvin Klein used the term techno-sexual in a 2007 campaign to promote a unisex fragrance called CK IN2U (Wilson, 2007). The advertising for CK IN2U conjured an edgy 'geek chic' and addressed the young, techno-savvy urbanite. According to the *New York Times*, the fragrance bottle was designed to remind con-sumers of the hi-tech iPod (Wilson, 2007). Calvin Klein set up a social networking website (*whatyouarein2.com* accessed 19 October 2007). A computer-generated advertisement in the style of the interactive game, *Second Life*, has appeared on *YouTube* (see: *youtube.com/watch?v=4y9vy-85Cfwg* accessed 10 August 2008). Media commentary has argued that the term technosexual is fake (Greenwood, 2007). But Calvin Klein has previously referred to marginal sexual meanings in their advertising, with great success. As Susan Bordo has pointed out, the publication of advertisements of Calvin Klein underwear featuring sinuous and beau-tiful male forms in the mid 1980s, marked changes in notions of desire and masculinity (1999). Those 1980s advertisements and their succes-sors are regarded as examples of the break from the tyranny of the so-called heteronormative male gaze through their appeals to hetero-sexual women and gay men. A recent article in the *Sydney Morning Herald* concerning sexuality and relationships made reference to metro-, retro-

and technosexuality (Brett, 2006). In this case, technosexual applied to men was seen as disparaging, like the apparently vain and effete, metrosexual. Such uses of technosexual raise questions concerning the contestation of desires and identities in the media-saturated late modern condition of urban sophisticates. In the marketing of CK IN2U, technosexuality trades on the sexual connotations of the internet and mobile telephony. Technosexual is meant to signify the potent mingling of emerging technological capacities and sexual and romantic desire. Like Calvin Klein underwear advertisements and terms such as retro- and metro-sexuality, technosexuality also provides a way of addressing sexual alterity, permitting reference to sexual and romantic life that exists outside of heteronormative domestic existence. Technosexuality is therefore also a method of offering up sexual alterity to forms of commercial exploitation. Adam Arvidsson has made a similar argument in an analysis of personal profiles posted to *Match.com* (2006). Arvidsson argued that e-dating is a prime example of the information economy, which is focused on the branding of social knowledge and, in the case of e-dating and other forms of internet-mediated partnering, social relations. Technosexuality as trademark attaches commercial enterprise to the technological articulations of sexual desire, romantic longing and partnering. *MySpace* and *Facebook* can be taken as other examples of the branding of internet-mediated social relations.

The Calvin Klein corporation is not alone in its fascination with technosexuality. An article in *The Futurist* magazine has speculated on the various ways that technologies will come to shape sexual practice (Garland, 2004). The article catalogued the technologies involved, including: the new media (internet); sexuopharmacy (Viagra); and the simulation of embodied experience, or haptics (computer-mediated sensory experience). Implicit in this story was the notion of innovation as the gradual accumulation of improved technological capacities and therefore an assumption that such progressive telescoping of technologies in the domain of sexuality is, on balance, a good thing. The article was positive in its outlook, asserting that technological developments will improve the experience of sex. This depiction of technological innovation therefore subscribes to a meta-narrative of modernisation: that the rational application of science and technology is good for society. In his book *The Digital Sublime: Myth, Power and Cyberspace* (2004), Vincent Mosco catalogued the different forms of communication technologies that have inspired both great hopes for the future of humankind and doom-saying. Mosco argued that such technological innovation is understood through myths of "... transcendent virtues" and "demonisation" (2004: 24). The article in *The Futurist* subscribed to the transcendent or utopian myth of technological innovation. The article did discuss the proliferation of cyber-pornography and questions over the loss of control over personal images published on the internet, but it did not explore the ways in which the internet can be used to further sexual exploitation, particularly of women and children. This limited, but positive outlook in the article was also expressed in relation to the depiction of sexual health. It seemed that technological innovation holds the promise of conquering sexually transmitted infections. In particular, it was argued that developments in telemedicine, home-testing kits for common infections, and the Do-It-Yourself logic of the internet may lead to the improved control of sexually transmitted infections.

Apart from questions of the cultural contest of desire intersecting with new technologies and the hopeful modernising of sexual health via technological innovation, there is evidence that people are using the internet in and around their intimate and sexual life in significant numbers. According to Arvidsson, nearly half of *Match.com* e-daters had met another e-dater offline (2006). Of those, 63% reported having sex with at least one person met online. An online survey of internet users (n=4500 approx.) conducted by researchers in the United States revealed that nearly half of the sample reported sex with internet partners (McFarlane et al., 2002). Canadian researchers have shown that nearly half their sample of university students (n=760) had used the internet to find information regarding sexual health (Boies, 2002). A survey of gay men and other homosexually active men living in England (n=2142) found that 66.2 per cent had used the internet to find a sex partner (Weatherburn et al., 2003). In contrast with these figures, but nevertheless lending support to the significance of internet-mediated sexual relating, a United States survey of people with internet access attending a sexual health clinic (n=2159) found that 6.8 per cent reported having sex with someone they had met online (Rietmeijer et al., 2003).

Research has also begun to document the dystopian aspects of technosexuality. There are examples of cyber-stalking and other forms of mediated harassment perpetrated by men, sometimes networks of men, on women (Adam, 2001; Philips & Morrissey, 2004). The internet has been implicated in the extension of the sexual exploitation and trafficking of women and children (Hearn, 2006; Long, 2004). The widespread phenomenon of the production and circulation of pornographic images through the internet is said to be a prime example of the negative impact of the internet on sexual practice (Fisher & Barak, 2001). Articles in *The Age* (Melbourne) argued that cyber-pornography leads to the breakdown of relationships (Horin, 2007). Internet pornography was likened to the advent of the Pill in the sexual lives of heterosexual couples, but in a way that contributed to marriage breakdown. It was argued through the concept of addiction that men can become so compulsive in their consumption of pornographic online images that they forgo sexual intercourse or, probably much worse, try to emulate the pornography they consume. So worrisome is the internet for intimate life that internet-related infidelity has become a focus for family therapy (Hertlain & Piercy, 2006) and social research (Whitty & Carr, 2006). Dating websites carry soothing words of advice and pop psychology tips for those worried about the online sexual activity of their partners. In addition, the internet age has seemingly ushered in new forms of cyber-sexual pathology (Cooper et al., 1999). As Anthony Pryce has pointed out, the interrogation of cybersex addiction discourse is a worthy topic for a book in its own right (2008).

As I have suggested, the notion of technosexuality can be extended to Viagra and related products. Annie Potts, among others, has for some time now investigated the social aspects of Viagra in the sexual lives of men and women (Potts & Tiefer, 2006). Dating from around the time of the introduction of Viagra itself in 1998, this scholarship maps the rise of this formation of technosexuality, providing a sustained and theoretically sophisticated exploration of the various aspects of the phenomenon. This work is revealing a paradoxical medicalisation and de-medicalisation of the sexual bodies of men and women. It is also suggesting the importance of the internet-mediated circulation of bio-technological knowledge, effects and products in sexual relating and experience.

Sexuality, technology and public health

It does seem possible to argue for the emergence of kinds of techno-sexuality comprised of bio- and communication technologies, sexual interests, market possibilities, hopeful rationalisation of sexual health, but also concerns over the kinds of technosexual subjects we may become. Public health intersects with these technosexual forms in terms of concerns over health risks, and the exploitation of technosexuality in efforts to further health care. Although changing, it appears also that public health research exhibits a prioritisation of, or even bias towards, gay men and young people in the affluent countries of Northern Europe, North America and Australasia. Public health is itself heavily reliant on technology and as with other aspects of late modern life, is being transformed by technological developments. But it is also the case that public health rationalities give sexual technologisation some of its logic.

Bio-technologies can be applied to the management of sexual health in a direct sense. For example, the female condom is regarded as a technological solution for women trying to reduce their risk of sexually transmitted infections and HIV (Kaler, 2004). Vaginal microbicide gels that inhibit HIV transmission are being trialled as methods of HIV prevention (Joglekar et al., 2007). The attempts to use circumcision as a method of HIV prevention could be taken to be bio-technological interventions (Imrie et al., 2007). HIV treatment can also be used to inhibit infection for example, in the birth process from mother to baby (Etiebet et al., 2004), following needle-stick injuries, and after an episode of sex without condoms (Korner et al., 2006).

In addition to bio-technology, public health has become attracted to the internet as a medium for intervention. Indeed, the internet is being heavily exploited in health care in general. *NHS Online* and *NHS Direct* are examples of state operated new media services in the United Kingdom (Nettleton & Hanlon, 2006). A United Kingdom website (*dipex.org* accessed 10 August 2008) publishes personal narratives regarding various diseases, including cancer and HIV. The website is seen as a method for sensitising health-care practitioners to the lived experience of people with illness. Researchers have argued that HIV stories published on the internet are therapeutic for people with HIV infection (Mohammed & Thombre, 2005). Another United Kingdom website (*livingstories.org.uk* accessed 10 August 2008) has published the stories of people living with haemophilia and HIV with the aim of drawing attention to the psychosocial needs and achievements of a group of people somewhat ignored in public policy.

Internet-based interventions for sexual health are proliferating on a global scale. The internet and other media in the United States have been used to address sexual health concerns among African American and Hispanic women (Anderton & Valdiserri, 2005). Online sex education websites for young people have been developed in the United States (Gilbert et al., 2005), China (Lou et al., 2006) and South Africa (Mitchell et al., 2004). Public health practitioners are advocating the use of internet cafes as a means of promoting access to sexual and reproductive health resources for women of all ages in Africa (Pillsbury & Mayer, 2005). The internet is also regarded as important for sexual health care among gay men in Australia (Murphy et al., 2004), the United Kingdom (Weatherburn et al., 2003) and the United States (Rhodes, 2004).

In addition to such innovations, some uses of the internet extend public health in controversial ways. According to an article in *HIV Plus*, an information magazine for people with HIV and their advocates, public health practitioners in the United States have used emails to conduct contact tracing among gay men who may have been exposed to syphilis (Adams, 2004). Contact tracing is a public health approach to disease control. When someone comes to a clinic and is found to have an infection, they may be asked to provide the names and contact details of their sex partners so that those people can also be tested and treated for the infection. According to the article, gay men use the internet to find sex partners, but in many instances, the names and contact details of these partners are not known. Such lack of information means that these men cannot be contacted in the usual way by letter or telephone. Apparently, public health practitioners have resorted to using online dating email systems to contact men and ask them to have tests for syphilis. Commentators have pointed out that this method of contact tracing raises concerns regarding consent and the mis-direction of contact tracing emails. However, public health practitioners seem undeterred. In a review of the development of online interventions, researchers have identified how these could be used to encourage testing for HIV, for partner notification, and as a medium for behaviour change interventions (Rietmeijer & Shamos, 2007).

But public health is not simply applying technology to the management of sexually transmitted infections and HIV. It also works to bring forms of technosexuality into existence by forming connections between technological systems implicated in sexuality with those that are salient for public health governance. These connections are also somewhat ambiguous, apparently furthering the institutional power of public health, but also de-centring its authority through the notion of the self-determining patient/consumer. An example is the 'Safe Sex Passport' (*safesexpassport. com* accessed 15 January 2008). This United States website, apparently allowed users of e-dating websites, and presumably other forms of online interaction, to record online the results of their tests for sexually transmitted infections. Potential e-dates were given an access code that allowed them to find out the subscriber's test results. In addition, public health practitioners have advocated that e-dating websites should include sexual health descriptor fields in online profiles so that e-daters can indicate their health status, that is: "... date of last STD screening, HIV serostatus, and genital herpes or genital wart history" (Levine & Klausner, 2005: 55). Both these strategies express a long-standing approach to the avoidance of sexually transmitted infections and HIV. In interviews with hetero-

sexual men regarding sexual intercourse and HIV risk, Waldby and colleagues argued that the interviewees relied on notions of women as
either clean or unclean (1993). Such notions were said to represent a
'cordon sanitaire' rationality used by heterosexual men to select sexual
partners. Waldby and colleagues noted:

> ... we would argue that their use of the clean/unclean dichotomy
> derives quite directly from the explanatory logic of most contem-
> porary HIV/AIDS education programs addressed to heterosexuals,
> which after all share the same history of ideas. They rely on the div-
> ision regularly made between 'the general population' and 'risk
> groups' (1993: 37).

Strategies such as the Safe Sex Passport and attempts to use e-dating
profiles to exhibit sexual health status, draw on, and help to make
literal, notions of cordon sanitaire, clean/unclean, and the avoidance
of risk groups. Aside from questions over utility as methods of public
health governance, the examples of the Safe Sex Passport and sexual
health descriptor fields show how a public health rationality can be
taken into, and give shape to, forms of online relating. In contrast,
internet-based forms of mediated health care can also de-centre authority and give rise to the prospect of the autonomous consumer in public
health. As I have indicated, Viagra and related products appear to be
implicated in such processes. Fox and Ward have pointed out in their
research concerning Viagra and other pharmaceutical products, that
the internet is now replete with websites, interactive forums and e-mail
lists that allow people to share information and advice (2006). In discussion forums for Viagra, participants write stories regarding their
experiences and circulate strategies for accessing and using the product. Fox and Ward also document the existence of e-clinics which
allow users to assess their own suitability for Viagra. Similarly, there are
websites that allow users to assess the extent of their risk for HIV infection, based on their responses to questions (*see vpul.upenn.edu/ohe/library/
Sexhealth/hiv/risassessment.htm and thebody.com/surveys/sexsurvey.html*,
both accessed 10 August 2008). Whether furthering or de-centring medical
and public health authority, such uses of the internet reveal how the
medical and public health logics of diagnosis, prescription and risk assess-
ment are able to be translated into the systems of coding and data pro-
cessing that constitute information technology.

Public health has also come to regard technologies implicated in sexual
practices as sources of risk for sexually transmitted infections and HIV. As

with other areas of sexual health, young people and gay men appear to be the focus of this activity. For example, my Medline search of articles concerning sexual health and the internet for the period 2000 to 2007 produced seven articles concerning gay men and 21 concerning young people (another nine addressed a mixture of concerns including an emergency contraception website and the use of the internet by patients attending sexual health clinics). It has been argued that young adults who use the internet to find sex partners are at risk of sexually transmitted infections (McFarlane et al., 2002). The internet has also been considered as a risk for transmission of HIV among gay men (Bolding et al., 2005). Researchers have considered if the implications of effective HIV treatment on HIV transmission have led gay men to give up using condoms (Elford & Hart, 2005). Viagra has also made an appearance as a possible risk for sexually transmitted infections and HIV among gay men (Halkitis & Green, 2007) and heterosexual men (Fisher et al., 2006). This interest in whether bio- and communication technologies are associated with risk for the transmission of sexually transmitted infections and HIV relies on a form of determinism that sets technology above other influences on sexual practice. I will show in the coming chapters that determinist assumptions regarding technosexuality are not particularly useful, but continue to frame understandings of internet-based and other technological mediations of sexual practice.

The bias towards gay men in social research regarding technosexuality reflects the extent to which they have been affected by HIV and other sexually transmitted infections and also that such men are now understood to use the internet for sexual purposes more than other groups. But it is also the case that a moral panic has contributed to this research, questioning the outward justification of public health need. In this regard there has been a flurry of media stories concerning 'barebacking' among gay men who use the internet to find sexual partners. Barebacking has various definitions, but in general, refers to intentional anal sex without condoms that may transmit HIV (Mansergh et al., 2002). This is a contentious issue that I will consider in more detail in the chapters to come. But for present purposes it is enough to record that a judgemental discourse has arisen that focuses on the supposedly reprehensible ethical failures of so-called barebackers. In his book, *What do gay men want?*, David Halperin argued that barebacking research reflects a turning back to notions of homosexuality as psychological dysfunction (2007). A review of sex education websites, found only three of 21 sites referred to gay men (Noar et al., 2006). The remainder focused on the sexual health of young people. On that basis, the authors called for increased attention to the sexual health of gay men in online sexual health care. In light of Halperin's argument, the call for more attention to the sexual practice of gay men could be seen to be a variation on the theme of psychopathologisation. However, it seems that a dominant concern for public health practitioners is the sexual health of young people. We could argue therefore that gay and other homosexually interested men suffer heightened scrutiny of their technosexual behaviour, but are not also provided commensurate online resources. This hyper-scrutiny of errant sexual practices and lack of services represents another variation on Halperin's thesis of pathologisation. In this view, the general shape of public health governance works to form a kind of positive production of sexual (ill)health among gay men by focusing on their supposed failures, without properly addressing their needs.

Defining public health

It appears that public health governance is exercised on and through, forms of technosexuality, at times relying on notions of cordon sanitaire and technological determinism. This book is concerned with such approaches and assumptions in public health governance. But it is necessary to be clear at the outset how I will use the concept of public health governance. It would be easy to use the terms public health and sexual health interchangeably in an analysis of sex, technology and public health, particularly in a focus on sexually transmitted infections and HIV. But I want to make a separation between public health governance and sexual health. For the present argument, I assume that public health is a form of governance that addresses the goal of sexual health. Public health is a wide range of activities, knowledge systems and institutional practices addressing the good health of citizens at large. Sexual health can be taken to be one aspect or aim of this general mode of public health governance. Sexual health care has specific features, but it relies on, and informs, public health governance. I want to keep both public health and sexual health in play in this book because I think that technosexuality has implications that go beyond sexual health care. Sexual health itself is subject to a tension concerning the relationship between disease and social justice models of practice. The disease model emphasises the eradication of disease, while the social justice model emphasises sexual enjoyment and wellbeing, the cultural aspects of sexuality, and citizenship. I want to recognise this tension as a source for critical inquiry regarding the public health governance of technosexuality.

There is good reason to address public health as a form of governance. As Petersen and Lupton have pointed out, public health is not easy to reduce to a definition (1996). Many forms of social action can be taken to comprise public health, for example: legislative change; policy work; environmental interventions; research; health education and health promotion; and orienting clinical services to detect, treat and prevent illness. Public health is also somewhat eclectic, drawing on: biological science; health technologies; epidemiology; and the social sciences. Public health cannot be easily located in terms of institutional context. For example, government and non-government agencies, the media, education, and the hospital system are all involved in public health action. However, there is an underlying imperative that joins up these activities, forms of knowledge and institutions. This imperative concerns the need to address population health through the action of individual citizens. The new public health as it has been called, makes this imperative explicit by addressing the psychological, social and cultural aspects of the health behaviour of the individual as the means of achieving the eradication and moderation of disease. This imperative also translates into a form of public health that embraces civil society through its constituent citizens. As Petersen and Lupton pointed out: "... everyone is, to some extent, caught up within what has become an expanding web of power and knowledge around the problematic of public health" (1996: 6). Public health is therefore necessarily a form of governance that addresses social goals via notions of citizenship. This book is concerned with the relationship between citizens and the social good articulated through public health governance of technologies that have implications for sexually transmitted infections and HIV. When I refer to public health in this book I mean the discursive expression of the assumptions, rationalities, conceptual frameworks and imperatives that join up research accounts, institutional practices of government and non-government agencies, media stories regarding technosexuality and sexual health, and personal experience narratives regarding technosexuality.

I also assume that sexual health is one aim of such public health governance. However, sexual health itself is defined in several ways that differ according to the emphasis placed on pleasure. Sexual health can be defined narrowly as the absence of disease or, more inclusively, as a form of social justice. The narrow disease model focuses on the control of infectious diseases through medical and behavioural interventions

(Coveney & Bunton, 2003). This focus is typically the work of local clinical services. In general, community, national and international health agencies subscribe to a notion of sexual health that embraces social justice. The World Association for Sexual Health (*worldsexology. org* accessed 10 August 2008) and the World Health Organisation (*who.int* accessed 10 August 2008) share a notion of sexual health as more than absence of disease and encompassing universal rights enshrined in international laws related to: autonomy; freedom of association; freedom from coercion and violence; and access to knowledge and education, reproductive decision-making, sexual health care. In addition, public health and sexual health can be distinguished according to how each articulate with pleasure. Public health discourse does not normally concern itself with sexual pleasure. Sexual health defined in broad terms does regard sexual pleasure as an aspect of wellbeing and therefore rightly incorporated into its discourse and action.

This tension or incommensurability of public health and sexual health concerning pleasure has much to reveal of the governance of technosexuality. Researchers have argued that a narrow mode of sexual health pervades much of the research that has been conducted in relation to technosexuality (Weatherburn et al., 2003). The narrow disease model focuses on measures of association and linear pathways of cause and effect, for example, by correlating measures of risk behaviour with measures of internet use. The moral panic over seeking barebacking partners online is another example. Such an approach leads to a view of the internet and sex as a danger for sexual health and obscures the positive aspects of the technology in sexual life. As Peter Weatherburn and his colleagues have pointed out (2003), if sexual health is defined to incorporate pleasure, the internet emerges as a technology for the enhancement of sexual experience and on that basis, a useful method for the promotion of sexual health.

The social justice model of sexual health also articulates with notions of sexual citizenship. Richard Parker has made the point that the sexual health as social justice movement has come from the margins of medicine (2007). Genito-urinary medicine clinics, reproductive health agencies, gay and lesbian communities, and women's health movements count among the originators of the idea of sexual health as a form of social justice. Such movements have sustained a dynamic but fragile dialogue of disease control and social justice. Parker has argued that it is not possible to address sexual health by focusing on the biological characteristics of the individual alone. Poverty, violence, gender power, stigma, discrimination, ageism all influence the vulnerability of the person. Parker has written of the need for a "... socially engaged agency" to properly address sexual health (2007: 973). In this line of argument, "... true sexual citizenship is contingent on the articulation of social justice in the area of sexuality" (2007: 973). This definition of sexual health in general translates into a vulnerability approach to action that focuses on inequalities in gender power, service reorientation and development, and addressing unequal access to education and sexual health care (WHO, 2006). Practitioners have made explicit links between sexual health, citizenship and human rights discourse and applied these to address the domination of women and marginalisation of gay men, but also, the imperatives of masculinity placed on heterosexual men (Liguori & Lamas, 2003).

It would be a mistake, however, to assume that the disease model should be ignored in preference for social justice. Instead, we need to draw on the tension between them as a foundation for critical inquiry in the area of technosexuality and beyond. Feminist researchers have argued against formalising definitions of health in general, and by extension, sexual health. For example, Laura Purdy has argued that notions of health defined in terms of wellbeing may work to extend forms of medicalisation, by furthering the inclusion of social practices into the oversight of medicine (2001). In this view it may be that it is better to have no definition of sexual health as such. Monica Greco has argued that the erosion of the boundary between "artificial/social" that is being achieved through bio-technology (2004: 7) makes the biological model of disease itself a political domain, replete with questions of democracy and social justice. For Greco, addressing health now requires:

> ... a new politics and ethics that self-consciously value the artificiality of human existence and that creatively appropriate the potential for choice made available through technology ... we are already witnessing a pluralisation of norms of life and health, and the opening of such norms to democratic debate. (2004: 8)

Similarly, in his work on the new genetics, Nikolas Rose is adamant that bio-technological models of health and disease are engaged with as a matter of politics and ethics (2001: 22). These arguments imply that we need new frameworks of critical analysis that can address the political questions inherent in bio-technological models of health and disease. These arguments also imply that both disease and social justice models need to be carefully appraised in terms of their political and social effects.

Technosexual citizenship?

Technosexuality has become interesting to public health governance both in terms of its supposed dangers but also in terms of possibilities for intervention. At the heart of this government of technosexual risks and possibilities are questions concerning the kinds of technosexual citizens that are coming into being. Petersen and Lupton have argued that modern systems of public health governance address social actors as citizens (1996). Following Parker already discussed, sexual citizenship appears to have relevance for sexual health care (2007). Greco (2004) and Rose (2001) have articulated the political questions of biotechnology as citizenship. Sexual citizenship per se is a well-developed literature. Several authors have used the concept of citizenship to address sexuality in late modern times, through such concepts as: 'intimate citizenship' (Plummer, 2003); 'sexual citizenship' (Weeks, 2007); and 'intimate democracy' (Giddens, 1992). Sexual citizenship has been used to consider the governance of sexual practice (Waites, 2005) and the effects of biomedical definitions of sexual difference (Epstein, 2003). In general, the notion of sexual citizenship addresses the gathering importance of reflexivity with regard to intimate and sexual life, and therefore, the new life politics regarding intimacy and sexual practice. While it has been recognised that technosexuality has implications for this new life politics (Plummer, 2003; Weeks, 2007), few have addressed technosexuality with reference to citizenship in a sustained way. This book goes some way to address this gap and assess the value of the citizenship perspective for interrogating public health and its engagements with technosexuality.

The notion of citizenship in general is closely associated with the political philosophy of the modern period. Citizenship can be defined as the combination of civil, political and social rights and responsibilities that provide the conditions of individual and collective existence (Giddens, 1992). Examples of citizenship rights and responsibilities include, universal suffrage, laws concerning gender and ethnic equality, social justice and so on. The sexuality and citizenship perspectives are seen to have a mutually productive relationship. Sexuality extends questions of citizenship to include the intimate, sexual relations of the private sphere. The concept of citizenship helps foreground the public implications of intimacy and sexual practice. Sexual citizenship therefore implies a life politics that traverses private and public spheres of social experience. It implies questions of relationality, that is, how individuals conduct their intimate relations. It is also a concept that draws attention to the ethical considerations of autonomy and constraint that have resonance with the models of sexual health I have discussed. For example, notions of freedom of association, freedom from coercion and the exercise of mutually satisfactory pleasure, form points of continuity between sexual health as social justice and the notions of sexual citizenship that appear in the literature.

However, technosexual citizenship has created only some academic interest. Such work is disseminated across various disciplines. Quite often, it operates by implication rather than explication, and, like critical studies of sexualities in general, is somewhat marginal. For example, search of new media journals and science and technology journals oriented to bio-technologies, shows that research regarding the sexual uses of technology remains marginal. As I have indicated, technosexual forms emerge in the public health literature, mainly as a danger for sexual health or as a way of extending interventions. Fortunately, some scholars have made sustained inquiries into aspects of technosexuality that do bear on questions of citizenship. Shelley Turkle's *Life on the screen: identity in the age of the Internet* (1997 [1995]), stands out as one of the first attempts to reflect on intimate, sexual relations and the internet. More recent cyber-ethnographic research pertaining to technosexuality has built on, or attempted to refute, Turkle's concepts, particularly in relation to what is seen as her optimism regarding the internet. Turkle's work remains central however, because of the commitment to detail and the prescience of many of the reflections on internet-mediated social and psychological experience. Waskul and colleagues have addressed cyber-pornography and related sexual uses of the internet, for example, in terms of how the market for pornography has sustained the internet, methods of its regulation, and internet-mediated sex work (2004). Another book by Waskul has explored identity and embodiment in relation to online sexual interaction, such as webcam sex (2003). The social psychology of internet-mediated dating has been described by Whitty and Carr in their book *Cyberspace Romance*, with particular reference to social cognition and online interaction, and following Turkle, the notion of erotic cyberspace as transitional space (2006). Working with a fusion of cultural studies and feminist philosophy of science, Luciana Parisi in her book *Abstract Sex* has created an account of technosex as informational, traversing bio- and information technologies at the level of molecules and bacteria (2004). Parisi documents the confusing proliferation of bio-info-technological forms of life which raise questions concerning the boundaries of nature and culture, but that also implicate human agency among other forms, inside the production of life. Parisi also makes an argument against the patriarchical fantasy of the domination of nature through culture. As I have noted, a critical feminist literature has addressed sexuopharmacy such as the introduction of the contraceptive Pill (Cook, 2005) and Viagra (Potts & Tiefer, 2006). Claudia Springer has made the point that technological innovations of the industrial and information age have often acquired sexual and gendered meanings (1996). A key motif in Springer's argument is the robot in the 1927 film *Metropolis*. The robot is both alluring and threatening, providing a metaphorical figure for utopian/dystopian cultural engagements with technological innovation and its sexual connotations.

However, some scholarship is more explicitly concerned with technosexual citizenship. By drawing on the relationship between space and sexual identity in urban environments (for example, gay community spaces) and also the implications of cyberspace for its discipline, geographers have begun to reflect on sexual citizenship and the internet (Hearn, 2006). With reference to concerns such as cyberstalking, Alison Adam has provided an account of the implications of internet-based sociality for gender relations and, by implication, sexual citizenship (2001). Working with reference to popular culture and feminism, Feona Attwood has identified how new technologies impinge on the kinds of intimate and sexual relationships that are coming into being (2006). In their book *Techno-sexual Landscapes*, Gordo-Lopez and Cleminson have taken up the notion of technosexuality in terms of "... quotidian materiality" (2004: 111). Gordo-Lopez and Cleminson were members of the University of Bradford, Sexuality and Technology Research Group (1996–7). They made an argument that technological innovation has long had connotations of sin and desire that sponsored questions of good government. They used examples as diverse as the sex segregation of the monasteries and the mills of the medieval period and the sexual implications of the railways of the industrial age. Gordo-Lopez and Cleminson also referred to the ways in which J.G. Ballard's 1973 book *Crash,* and the 1995 film of the same name, depicted the pleasure that could be extracted from the bloody fusion of bodies and machines in car crashes, both accidental and deliberate. The film in particular led to controversies regarding censorship. The subject of the book and film therefore mobilised questions of sexual pleasure, technology and governance, serving as flashpoints in the history of technosexual citizenship. These authors also pointed to the necessary engagement with questions of technosexuality and citizenship because of the rise of both the internet and bio-technologies:

> ... it is important to understand the increasing interest in computer-mediated sexual encounters and relations, for instance, in 'safe' textual and virtual spaces. These new textual exchanges in the Net contrast, it would seem, with the return of biological accounts of sexual identity as indicated by the popularity of neurogenetic research into the biological basis of sexual preference. Furthermore, this return of biological accounts of the social is accompanied by a new technologisation of material and sexual matters. This is a phenomenon that brings a paradoxical outcome. There may be increased medical intervention in the field of the body but the individual apparently enjoys greater flexibility from shaping the individual body (piercing, tattoos and plastic surgery). (2004: 107–108)

Gordo-Lopez and Cleminson have therefore pointed to the simultaneous mediatisation and bio-technologisation of sexual practice and a double movement of expanding options for the manipulation of the sexual body and relations, with an intensification of bio-technological understandings of sexuality. The intersection of technosexuality and public health governance, with all its associations with both bio- and communication technologies and its requirements on good citizens, is an especially apt example of Gordo-Lopez and Cleminson's thesis.

Overview

The old relationships between sexuality, technological change and the governance of civil society are finding expression in such technosexual forms as e-dating and Viagra use. The mixing of bio- and communication technologies appears to be a significant, if not axiomatic, aspect of technosexuality. Public health has been quick to seize on such techno-sexual practices as a source of the endangerment of healthy sexuality but also as the means to intervene in the lives of technosexual citizens. This book concerns itself with these relationships between sex, technology and governance with particular reference to the duality in public health that recognises in technosexuality both danger and the means for extending itself. For a project such as this, it is necessary to establish an account of technosexuality that permits interrogation of how it is being governed in public health. Some of this book is therefore devoted to drawing together research and scholarship regarding technosexuality. In particular, I will draw on scholarship that has considered technologies relevant to sexuality, sexual citizenship studies, and public health itself. A key theme in this elaboration of a social theory of technosexuality will be the self-awareness implied in questions of citizenship. As I will discuss, technosexuality necessarily raises the ethical question: 'How shall I be technosexual?'. This question derives from the more general one of 'How shall I be?', that, according to many theorists of self and society, is at the centre of reflexive modernisation (see for example: Giddens, 1991). Such questions resonate with the ethical considerations of bio- and communication technologies noted by Gordo-Lopez and Cleminson, Greco, Rose and many others. As I will argue, public health governance also asserts itself through such questions of ethical being.

It is also important to recognise what this book will not do. As will have become plain in the previous discussion, there are many possible implications of the connections between sexuality and technology. So there is some terrain that this book cannot address. For instance, this book does not consider in any depth the important areas of reproductive health technologies and internet-based sexual exploitation and pornography. The book is also delimited by a focus on the ways technologies mediate and inform sexual relations that have implications for sexually transmitted infections and HIV. I am not therefore going to dwell on virtual sex, 'tiny sex' as it is called in online game environments (Turkle, 1997 [1995]), or the far-flung cybersex networks of the internet (Waskul, 2003; Waskul, 2004). I am not going to address the sex-technology connection through the concept of addiction (Cooper et al., 1999), except to make a critical argument concerning the unsatisfactory determinism circulating in some such views of sexuality and technology.

On the basis of a theoretically informed account of technosexuality, I want to reflect on public health governance with three main purposes in mind. The first concerns how public health conceptualises social action in relation to technosexual practices that have implications for sexually transmitted infections and HIV. In this regard, I want to consider how the imperatives of public health are brought into connection with notions of technological innovation, such as those that are in evidence in technosexuality. Second, and as I have indicated in the previous discussion, some of the assumptions concerning technosexual actors in public health research appear to over-determine the contribution of the technologies themselves. My argument will dispute crude forms of technological determinism, but equally, will critically appraise accounts of technosexuality that underestimate the capacities and influences of the internet and bio-technologies. As a way of addressing some of its assumptions, I want to retain the tension between techno- and cultural determinism in public health governance. For example, it is often argued that the anonymous character of online communication is the source of harm. In this book, I will argue for something quite different. I want to say that under public health governance, the technological mediations of intimate and sexual life provide methods for revealing identities, intentions, and practices, and that, contrary to much thought in this domain, there is good reason to argue that a common ethic of online social interaction concerns the transparency of self. The third main purpose of this book concerns a consideration of the mixing of bio- and communication technologies in techno-sexuality. I think there is much to be gained from exploring the ways in which bio- and communication technologies combine in techno-sexuality. I am not alone in emphasising such interconnections. For example, it has been argued that both bone densitometry and the internet are information technologies because they each provide knowledge important to considerations of hormone replacement therapy for women (Green et al., 2006). Extending this approach to the topic of this book implies the interdependence of bio- and communication technologies in the mediation of sexual practices, and by extension, public health itself. A common approach to critical analysis would be that such bio-technological mediations help extend public health authority over technosexual citizens, or in other words, medicalise technosexuality. I will consider the value of such an argument. However, I also want to reflect on the idea that public health governance is itself being trans-formed through technosexuality, in ways that produce challenges to citizenship, but also opportunities for extending social justice.

The chapters that follow reflect the shape of the argument for this book. In Chapter 2, I outline the theories that contribute to a social theory for sexuality and technology. In particular, I will consider the self-aware internet user, the notion of cyborg life, and connections with perspectives derived from the literature regarding sexual citizen-ship. The main purpose of this chapter is to critically reflect on the legacy of previous analysis and to determine a language for the book. In Chapters 3 and 4, I present two case studies. The first of these con-cerns internet-mediated partnering and sexual health. The second con-cerns the 'hyper-technologisation' of sexual practice produced by the mingling of internet-mediated partnering and the knowledge concern-ing HIV embodiment generated by bio-technologies. These two cases draw on published research, some of which I have written singly, or with the assistance of colleagues, in relation to the internet (in press; 2004; 2006b; 2006c) and HIV bio-technologies (2002; 2007; 2008; 2006a; 2002). In Chapters 5, 6 and 7, I address the implications of the technological mediations of sexual life for public health governance. In Chapter 5, I consider the major imperatives of public health and how they are applied to technological innovations. In this regard, I will consider altruism, contagion, and risk, including its forensic turning. This chapter will make an argument that public health is itself multiple, or even somewhat incoherent, because of its reliance on different imperatives. In Chapter 6, I will develop the concept of the technological mediations of visibility. With reference to moral panic concerning the technologisation of sexual cultures and what I have referred to elsewhere as spectacular risk (Davis, in press), I want to consider how forms of technosexuality serve public health governance. Chapter 7 considers more general questions of the public health governance of technosexuality with reference to debates concerning medicalisation, changes in medical authority, and the rise of the patient/consumer. The concluding chapter will summarise and reflect on the argument. As we will see in the chapters to follow, the public health governance of technosexuality is significant not only because of its implications for the intimate and sexual lives of citizens in late modern times, but also because it suggests a pattern for the governance of technologically-mediated society in general.

2
Technologies and Sexual Citizenship

Technosexuality is commonly understood as both dangerous and transcendent. There are many examples in popular culture that reinforce this duality. For example, in the 1992 film *The Lawnmower Man*, a powerful new computer technology is invented that enables full body virtual experience. A human who is literally attached to the technology takes on its capacities, becoming at first intelligent, but eventually a monster. In one segment of the film, the man and his woman partner have a virtual erotic experience, depicted in the form of computer-generated images of them embracing against a background of swirling colour. Their bodies become joined in the image of a beautiful, iridescent creature. The episode ends badly however. The film is not absolutely clear, but it implies a sexual assault on the woman by her partner. The interaction so portrayed is meant to imply that computer technology promises transcendent erotic experience. Virtual sexual space is understood as shapeless and given over to pleasure that has no limit. But, the assault is meant to suggest that desire, and in this instance, male heterosexual desire, has an instinctual, volatile basis and that technology has the power to bring it forth in a dangerous form. The reliance on these ideas of sex and technology makes it seem inevitable that men will lose control of themselves. This particular depiction of technosex also reveals a curiosity with new technology expressed through a resort to sexual meanings. It is as if the makers of the film relied on sexual desire as the best way of expressing the transcendent, but ultimately dangerous, capacity of computer technology.

The Lawnmower Man looks outdated in our own era of post-millennial technosexuality. But the example is not so different to more recent engagements with technosexuality. *The Lawnmower Man* suggests the deeply inscribed cultural understanding of technological innovation as both dangerous and transcendent. It also suggests that instinctual sexual desire itself is the most primitive human element that conjures the limit power of the implications of technological innovation for human life. High technology is thus opposed to sexual instinct to form an unpredictable confrontation of technological achievement and desire, raising questions concerning the kinds of beings we are to become. Although less sensational, the idea that internet-mediated sexual practices might be a danger for sexual health, but also an innovative method for extending public health interventions, refers to this pattern of danger and transcendence. It is necessary to recognise the traces of such notions in current engagements with technosexuality. It is also necessary to move beyond these notions to furnish the basis for a critique of public health governance. For these reasons, this chapter draws on relevant social theory and debate to develop a conceptual framework for technosexuality.

This chapter will take up the task of developing a conceptual framework for technosexuality based on two assumptions. The first of these has to do with sexuality as a matter of ethics in connection with the notion of reflexive modernisation. Authors such as Beck and Beck-Gernsheim and Giddens have argued that sexuality, and related concepts such as gender, love, intimacy, and sexual pleasure are subject to the de-traditionalising processes of modernity (Beck & Beck-Gernsheim, 1995; Giddens, 1992). Others have argued that sex and sexuality are now subject to what is called liquid modernity, a perspective which emphasises the evanescence of social bonds in the late modern order (Bauman, 2003). Plummer has written about the rise of multiple speaking positions in matters of sexual identity "… as the dominant meta-narrative gets fractured, dispersed or even eliminated" in the late modern era (1995: 142). These perspectives underline the dissolution of the universal ordering of sexuality in late modern times. Such changes have created new questions concerning how individuals should conduct themselves as sexual subjects. Technosexuality is one expression of this imperative on ethical sexual subjectivity, as writers such as Plummer (2003) and Weeks (2007) have noted.

The second important assumption I will rely on concerns the relationship between society and technology. In *Network Society*, Manuel Castells suggested that the effects of information technology cannot be separated from the "… historical specificity of social practices" that produce them (Castells, 2000: 441). Beck and Beck-Gernsheim have written of the relationship between society and technology as a kind of spiral: "… technology may be seen as a spiral-like process. It appears as both the product and the instrument of social needs, interests and conflicts. Technology is effect and cause at the same time" (2002: 139). Broadly, Bruno Latour and those who follow him, argue that technologies can be considered as actors in their own right, a perspective that gives rise to what is called actor-network theory (van Loon, 2008). In this view, a proper analysis of the technology-society connection comes to focus on the assemblage of human actors, technological actors, institutional practices, political assumptions, and so on, that comprise technosocial systems. In combination, these perspectives imply that to understand technosexuality we need to avoid either techno- or cultural determinism. Others have adopted this assumption to address technosexuality. For example, Gordo-Lopez and Cleminson made the argument that the 'magical and demonic' motion of the machinery of mills and railways and their capacity to throw people together in new liminal spaces inspired forms of social repression that assured the sexual power of such technology (2004). Central in this argument was the notion that technosocial change, movement of people and machines, and unruly mixing, excite new questions of desire and therefore social regulation. According to them, railway stations in particular have special status because they mark the transition from pre- to industrial age society. Railways can be said to be technologies that enabled the control over time and space and the communication of people, goods and information. They were therefore early technologies of globalisation. The internet is also a globalising technology that raises questions of desire, communication, unruly mixing and therefore good government. Gordo-Lopez and Cleminson thus placed technological changes into social context, but at the same time, explored the social effects of technological changes. In research of the introduction of the contraceptive Pill in the United Kingdom, Hera Cook argued that previous accounts had been either technologically or culturally over-determined, that is, under and over-estimating the social dimensions of the introduction of the drug (2005). Cook's line of argument was that the Pill had the effect of breaking the link between sexual practice, fertility, and economics for women, with vast implications for heterosexual relations. Cook's account is useful because it recognised how technologies can help produce kinds of social relations, but without collapsing into techno-determinism.

This chapter therefore aims to provide a conceptual framework for technosexuality that acknowledges the centrality of questions of ethical citizenship, and without resorting to either techno- or cultural-determinism. I want to use two main devices to explore this terrain and to provide the basis for the discussion of sexual citizenship I want to make later in this chapter. The first of these is what I refer to as the 'questing avatar' derived from the cyber-ethnographic research regarding the internet, intimacy and sexuality. An avatar is the, often personalised, graphic image of characters used in online interactive games, such as *Second Life*. I use this term questing avatar to summarise the project of self that can arise in online social experience. I also use this notion of the questing avatar to draw attention to notions of self-aware social action and technology. The second device I want to exploit is the Viagra cyborg, a term used by Annie Potts to refer to the mixing of human and pharmaceutical products in and around aspects of sexual embodiment (2005). Critical inquiry regarding sexuopharmacy has drawn attention to some of the other concerns of technosexuality regarding sexual embodiment, medicalisation and re-medicalisation, and the involvement of commercial activity in the production and exploitation of technosexual forms, such as the Viagra cyborg. My strategy of exploring these two devices provides an introduction to some of the most salient social theories for this investigation of technosexuality. But my main purpose is to draw on these notions of the questing avatar and the Viagra cyborg to identify and discuss some of the questions of ethics that arise in technosexuality and how these can be taken into a discussion of technosexual citizenship. It is important to bear in mind that I am using these technosexual figures to draw attention to two main themes in the extant literature and to provide the basis for exploring implications for citizenship. Not everyone will find themselves to be one or the other of these technosexual figures, although from time to time some of us may encounter questing avatars and Viagra cyborgs. In this discussion, I take these figures to be heuristic devices.

In the next sections, I develop these notions of questing avatars and Viagra cyborgs, with particular reference to the ethics of technosexual practice. In the following section, based on observations regarding the importance of reciprocal relations in online life and the social relations implied in sexuopharmacy such as Viagra, I develop a conceptualisation of technosexual citizenship that gives emphasis to relational ethics. I will make this argument with reference to debate regarding citizenship and also research that has employed citizenship perspectives to address sexually transmitted infections and HIV.

Questing avatars

The internet provides many examples of websites and communication practices that have sexual purposes. Along with the examples I mentioned in the previous chapter, there are websites where sex workers can market their services (Sanders, 2005). Sado-masochist websites exist (Palandri & Green, 2000) as do websites that provide travel and security advice for gay men who like cottaging (Ashford, 2006). There are international lesbian online communities (Burke, 2000) and communities for Japanese gay men and their admirers (McLelland, 2002). Such a kaleidoscope of technosexuality is hard to summarise in a way that can do justice to such diversity. But I do want to draw out a central theme that connects forms of technosexuality with social theory concerning reflexive modernisation and intimate life. In this regard I want to introduce the figure of the 'questing avatar' derived from the cyber-ethnographies of online intimate and sexual life. The term avatar comes from the world of online gaming. It is the visual representation of a game character. But as we shall see, avatars can do more than play games. They appear to take on social and psychological significance that have bases in the questions of self that are axiomatic for technosexual citizenship. In particular, online social interaction, particularly of the sexual kind, is deeply bound up with a quest for self-knowledge, and the necessary ethical relations of reciprocity and authenticity. It is my argument therefore that ethical conduct in relation to sexual relating is the method by which technosexuality comes into being. Citizenship does not arise outside or after technosexuality. Technosexuality is always already technosexual citizenship.

Though not altogether making commensurate arguments, several theorists have developed accounts of the late modern social order that pivot on the transformation of sexual and intimate life. Giddens has argued rather famously for the pure relationship and plastic sexuality (1992). He pointed to the love relationship as an end in itself as central to his theoretical development of reflexive modernisation. For Giddens, reflexive modernisation draws on his theory of structuration, where he argued that the self-aware agency of social actors both reproduces and modifies social structure. As he put it: "All forms of social life are partly constituted by actors' knowledge of them" (Giddens, 1990: 38). According to Giddens, partnering is no longer necessarily a reflection of economic necessity or tradition. Intimacy and sexual practice, so the theory goes, have become ends in themselves. Beck and Beck-Gernsheim adopt a similar approach centring on notions of de-traditionalisation and elective affinity (Beck & Beck-Gernsheim, 1995). They argue that in the pre- and early modern periods coupling was grounded in tradition, religious belief and economic strategies concerning the survival of the household. In the late modern period, partnering, for the most part, is predicated on love and desire between individuals who choose to be together primarily for the sake of the relationship itself. If any expectations exist for the intimate couple it is that they choose a life partner with whom they want to remain and for no other reason. Technosexuality could be taken to be exemplary reflexive transformation of intimate life. Because it foregrounds a self-aware social actor, internet-mediated partnering both reflects and helps to produce this late modern logic of sexual and emotional love as ends in themselves.

However, there is a possible contradiction or tension in this theory of reflexive intimacy that is relevant for technosexual citizenship. The idea of social agents freed from constraint implies that intimacy has less value in late modern society, or at least raises questions regarding its position in social relations. This is certainly an assumption that drives the idea that technosexuality is addictive and breaks down partnerships, as noted in Chapter 1. Some forms of public health also rely on this assumption to make arguments that technosexuality is a threat to sexual health. But, if intimacy is less important, how can it be that, as Arvidsson notes, perhaps nine million people subscribe to *Match.com* (2006)? Giddens deals with this contradiction by arguing that intimacy has, in fact, become *more* important in late modernity. The self-knowledge that an individual can acquire in the eyes of their loved one has taken central place in theories of self and society. For Giddens, the love bond is a source of ontological security for individuals facing the erosion of other grounds for a sense of self. For example:

> Erotic relations involve a progressive path of mutual discovery ... ... personal trust, therefore, has to be established through the process of self-enquiry: the discovery of oneself becomes a project directly involved with the reflexivity of modernity (Giddens, 1990: 122).

Giddens has also argued that such reflexive intimacy is the engine of what he refers to as intimate democracy (1992). He has suggested that reflexive intimacy enables the questioning of traditional gender relations, furthering egalitarian heterosexual partnering. However, the idea of the pure relationship has been criticised. For example, Jamieson has questioned whether women, and more particularly men, are interested in equality in their relationships, reflected in the continuing sexual division of labour in the domestic sphere (Jamieson, 2003). Giddens has acknowledged the idealisation that is implied in the idea of an intimate relationship as an end in itself (in particular, see Chapter 8t in *The Transformation of Intimacy*). Despite such controversy regarding the pure relationship, and as Giddens has pointed out, we can recognise that intimate life is important for the self and that it implies questions of, How shall I be?, or as in the present case, How shall I be technosexual?

The quest for self-knowledge through sexual relating is the central theme of one of the most famous cyber-ethnographies of online life. Shelley Turkle's engaging account of research in her 1996 book *Life on the screen: Identity in the age of the Internet,* helped establish cyber-ethnography, and provided a language for the relational and sexual aspects of cybersociety, and by implication, technosexual citizenship. Turkle focused on the culture of online games which involve multiple players. According to Turkle, such online interaction has sexual meaning, including, gender swapping and "netsex" or "... tiny sex" as it is referred to in online game environments (1997 [1995]: 21). In these games, people create avatars. In these environments it is possible to make one's avatar have tiny sex experiences, which involve instructing one's avatar to interact in a sexual way with another avatar, or several. Turkle was among the first to make the point that tiny sex is free from sexually transmitted infections and the need for contraception: "... virtual promiscuity never causes pregnancy or disease" (1997 [1995]: 208). This perspective sits in contrast with the notion that the internet may be harmful for sexual health.

However, the main theme of Turkle's argument concerned the ways in which online game players actively manipulate their self-presentations and reflect on the resulting social experiences. To make this argument regarding presentation of self and self-reflection, Turkle relied on psychoanalytic ideas of transitional objects and post-structural concepts of the fragmentation of identity. Turkle assumed that psychoanalysis is, at heart, a quest for self-knowledge. Because the online self is reflexively made, the imagination and emotions are deeply implicated in online social experience. In a banal sense, imagination is required to make online games work. There are cues in the graphics used to construct the game environments, but an ability to suspend disbelief is needed to experience and enjoy the game. In a more profound sense, being able to invest in the emotional life of an avatar requires a suspension of disbelief. But this emotional play reveals the self, or perhaps, promotes a confrontation with the self. In this regard, Turkle makes a parallel between the self work of online social interaction and the self work of psychoanalysis. As Turkle put it:

> Virtuality need not be a prison. It can be a raft, the ladder, the transitional space, the moratorium, that is discarded after reaching

greater freedom. We don't have to reject life on the screen, but we don't have to treat it as an alternative life either. We can use it as a space for growth. Having literally written our personae into existence, we are in a position to be more aware of what we project into everyday life. Like the anthropologist returning home from a foreign culture, the voyager in virtuality can return to a real world better equipped to understand its artifaces (Turkle, 1997 [1995]: 207).

To strengthen her argument, Turkle referred to the example of a woman amputee interviewed for the research. According to Turkle, this interviewee reported that her avatar did not have a limb. On that basis, the interviewee explored romantic attachments online as an amputee, therefore gaining courage to do so offline. In another example, Turkle referred to a man who adopted the persona of the film star Katherine Hepburn in his online life. His experiences as an online screen goddess were brought into his offline self, apparently strengthening and extending his experience of himself as a man. Pryce has developed a similar perspective in relation to a cyber-ethnography of homosexually interested, heterosexual men (2008). For some of these men, cybersex provided the means for learning to practice same sex desire, and therefore, but not always, modifying self-identity and sexual practice. In contrast, writers have written of cybersex in a sceptical manner, directly criticising Turkle's apparent utopianism. For example, a psychoanalyst referred to his clinical research with spanking and other fetishists to argue that internet pornography is a defense against intimacy (Young, 2002). As with Turkle, the internet is seen as a place of imaginative possibility. The online exercise of sexual phantasies might foster psychic growth, but could also provide for the extension of destructive emotions.

Also addressing the reflexive aspects of technosexuality, Don Slater (1998) has conducted an ethnography of what he called the 'IRC sex pic' scene (IRC stands for internet relay chat). Slater revealed how, because of its technosocial features, the sex pic scene is regulated according to an ethics of reciprocal relations. The sex pic scene involves sharing sexually explicit images. The scene contrasts with other forms of online sociality such as interactive games, e-dating sites or social networking sites because it is comprised of fleeting reciprocal relations that enable the exchange of pics. There are few ongoing relationships as such. According to Slater, sex pic trading has sex-shop conventionality that in general conforms to a heterosexual male cosmology of sexual interests. Slater pointed out that the images themselves have no inherent value because they are so abundant and, because of digital technologies, infinitely reproducible. This combination of impermanence and abundance leads to a situation where users are said to be "... battling to solidify their evanescence" (1998: 97). Resonating with Giddens's notion of reflexive intimacy, Slater argues that the sex pic scene creates a challenge for participants concerning ontological security:

> ... participants are forever wavering between a dismissive, cynical stance bolstered by defensive strategies and postures, and a trusting stance bolstered by strategies designed to authenticate the other by giving them an increasingly reliable 'body'. In sum, the problem that is practically posed to IRC participants by the performative nature of on-line identity is simply, how can I trust or believe anyone or anything? How can I accept the other, or be myself accepted, as an ethical subject? (Slater, 1998: 105)

The challenge of making the internet work in this way leads on to questions of ethics and through those, technosexual citizenship. Slater argued that the scene is sustained through a mixture of commodity and gift exchange, where reciprocity is the key imperative. The sex pic scene is therefore sustained by the qualities of the social relations between strangers. Although he admits that it is not a perfect system of social relations, Slater argues that the sex pic scene is only possible through a system of ethical accountability, or as he put it, by using strategies "... to establish a sense of ongoing ethical sociality" (2002: 227). For example, sex pic traders develop "... strategies of authentication" that help them to stabilise the identities of the other and themselves (1998: 92). Slater also makes the central point that it is the ontological insecurity of the IRC environment that may explain its sexualisation. Because sexual desire is understood as revealing the truth of the person, its expression in online society helps to provide a kind of ontological essence through which social relations can be established. The dominance of male heteronormative assumptions regarding sexual desire presumably reflects the population of traders, but it is also an expression of the need to establish the ontology of the sex pic scene and therefore establish trading relations. On this basis, Slater argued against the utopian understanding of the internet as a limitless space, noting that: "... we should look to the normative orders that operate in cyberspace in order to explain the kinds of materiality that are in fact produced there" (2002: 228). According to Slater, the IRC sex scene is a delimited sex public achieved through conventional notions of male heteronormativity, a notion of sexual desire as a truth of the self, and the active social regulation of the trading networks. On this basis, Slater made the point that online society is deeply circumscribed by familiar forms of sexual difference and that this manner of governance is given force precisely because of anxiety regarding the challenge of giving shape and purpose to internet-mediated relations.

The work of Turkle and Slater suggests that online sexual interaction is necessarily a quest for self identity, achieved through an ethics of reciprocity. Authenticity is also an important aspect of such techno-sexual citizenship. The importance of authentic online relations is seen in Jonathan Marshall's cyber-ethnography of an academic mailing list used by people from different parts of the world, who at times moved to internet gaming environments to engage in 'netsex' (2003). The article included a download of the text of a netsex event. As with tiny sex, sexual interaction is conducted through text and commanding one's avatar to perform in certain ways. Like Slater and to some extent Turkle, Marshall noted that a major challenge for participants of online social environments is the problem of authenticity. Drawing on Foucauldian notions of confessional, truth and sex, Marshall argued that the sexual qualities of internet-based interaction are vital because they stabilise the online presence of social actors. The ontological value of sexual desire is underlined since sex is not the primary focus in these mailing lists, which were ostensibly for academic purposes. Marshall observed that a feature of the internet communication is that one does not have an online presence unless one creates it in some way. Online presence can disappear in the click of a mouse, a refresh of a screen, or a computer crash. In this sense, Marshall's work intersects with Slater's. There is an underlying ontological anxiety for participants that the self has to be imagined and maintained as a social and psychological being, but also as a technological achievement. Marshall noted: "Online society is primarily a society of personal relations, which must be continually cultivated and reforged in a relatively unstable and unclear environment" (2003: 244). This underlying imperative of online survival may explain the operation of the social networking spaces *Facebook* and *MySpace*. These more recent socio-technical environments emphasise a more durable self, portrayed through a profile webpage and images and texts, which partly overcome some of the problems of the disappearing online self. According to Marshall, gender is a crucial aspect of the self that comes into being in online society. It appears that when people construct avatars, the representation of gender is an important way of conferring identity. Online game environments permit participants to stress or even over-emphasise their avatar gender. However, over-exaggeration of gender raises questions of authenticity. An avatar that is made to be overly masculine or feminine can take on a monstrous quality that jeopardises its value as a representation of self, destabilising online social interaction. Approaching this problem of authenticity in another way in a cyber-ethnography of an online community, Denise Carter argued that friendships formed online develop outside the constraints of gender, race, age and other social characteristics (2005). However, such friendships were not completely fictional. Carter observed that authenticity is significant for sustaining friendships in online communities. In particular, individuals are expected to be truthful about themselves, although they can reveal such truths gradually and carefully. In addition, participants were aware that when friendships moved offline, deception is exposed. So, to permit possible fleshly friendship, revealing truth online is necessary. Arvidsson has made a similar argument in relation to the online profiles of *Match.com* (2006). According to Arvidsson:

> ... the dominant element of a large majority of the profiles surveyed here was what one would call an 'experiential ethic' of self-discovery, an orientation towards touching, revealing or sharing one's true self through open-hearted and intimate communication with others ... (2006: 680).

Reflecting on online sexual relating among gay and other homo-sexually interested men, Dowsett and colleagues have likewise argued that online sociality is subject to: "... reciprocity, responsibility and comportment" (2008: 129).

Viagra cyborgs

The notion of the questing avatar goes some way in helping us to understand the link between online life and sexuality. The previous examples have emphasised self-aware action in relation to the new forms of constraint and possibility that exist in online life. In these accounts, the quest for self-knowledge and therefore the ontological security of the self depends on an online ethics of reciprocity and authenticity. Technosexuality is evanescent and experimental, but unlike the science fiction depictions of cybersex as limitless, it is remarkably closely policed and conventional. Indeed, normative understandings of sexuality and gender appear to provide the basis for citizenship in the challenging circumstances of online relating. Implicit in technosexual citizenship therefore is a tension between its productive qualities and normative social categories. In this section, I want to extend this argument to bio-technologies. Drawing on the notion of the Viagra cyborg established by Potts (2005), I will argue that using Viagra and similar products to correct erectile dysfunction is a form of technosexuality that challenges normative social categories of identity, embodiment and social relations. In particular, the Viagra cyborg implies technological breaches, or even a reconfiguration, of sexual embodiment. Viagra also appears to be a form of bio-technology that helps decentre medical authority over sexuality, permitting both the rise of the reflexive consumption of bio-technology and the attachment of bio-technology consumers to systems of commercial production. Viagra consumption therefore appears to provide a pattern for the social relations of consumers, medical authority and commerce that has implications for technosexuality in general. I also want to use the figure of the Viagra cyborg to draw attention to the ways that the internet and bio-technology can hybridise. This hybridisation will be important to the argument I want to make in later chapters concerning public health engagements with technosexuality.

Some theorists have argued that bio- and communication technologies, among others, are changing what it means to be human. Technologies extend human capacities. For example the motor-car helps us travel long distances in a short period of time. Mobile phones allow us to communicate as we travel across the city. As I noted in Chapter 1, haptic technologies promise forms of computer-mediated sensory experience. But we can also argue that taken for granted technologies such as the motor-car and mobile phone extend human capacities, to create new hybrid forms of techno-human life. Many depictions of such cyborgs exist in popular culture, for example, in the *Matrix, Terminator,* and *Robocop* films. But there are deeper implications of the notion of the human cyborg concerning the status of human life in a technologising world. Donna Haraway argued that the boundary between human and 'other' has been blurred in three ways: human-machine; human-animal; human-informational (1991). Along with machine-human hybrids such as the motor-car already mentioned, xenotransplantation and genetic modification technologies have breached the boundary between human and other forms of life. The internet and related technologies have transformed our capacity to deal with large amounts of information and data. Because many of us use these technologies every day, we can no longer speak of life existing without technology. Extending the Haraway argument, Tim Jordan has argued that some information technologies are alive, collapsing the boundary of nature and culture (1999). For example, the automatic functions of software, viruses and worms, and artificial intelligence can be regarded as 'life', or at least raise questions of what life is.

The question over what it means to be human is often the underlying theme of science fiction stories regarding cyborg life. Perhaps the most famous of these is Mary Shelley's *Frankenstein*. One of the key themes of this story is the revenge of the Monster on Dr Frankenstein. The Monster becomes aware of its status as part human and part monster, creating an emotional crisis that turns into destruction, a kind of post-human anguish turned to rage. Likewise, Dr Frankenstein becomes aware that he has transgressed a universal ethical standard by animating the monster, bringing into being a creature that is both human and not. Part of this post-human anguish is the realisation of the passing of an accepted form of human life and its status as the foundation for ethical social relations. The narrative of the *Lawnmower Man* already discussed, follows the pattern of Shelley's *Frankenstein*.

The point of these examples is that post-human anguish cannot be eschewed, but needs to be addressed as the basis for improved ethical social relations in relation to technology and society. Bio-technology alters human life in ways that do not necessarily fit with pre-existing assumptions regarding life. Haraway asserted that we need to embrace these new forms of life precisely because they do challenge normative social categories. In this view, the moments of post-human anguish that have occupied monsters and monster-makers are important because they reflect challenges to ethical arrangements that are the basis of citizenship. According to Haraway, engaging with such moments holds the promise of a better social justice for a technologising world. Retaining a notional, pre-technology, human self does violence to how we now experience our lives. In addition, reluctance to engage with the notional human cyborg has the effect of inhibiting a political engagement with the actors that have brought it into being, such as biomedicine, industrial production and commercial interests. Of course, not everyone has been so impressed with these arguments. For example, Deborah Lupton has written in a sceptical way about the prospect of cyborg life, arguing that social existence is still very much tied to fleshly existence and that cyborg life remains marginal to human experience (1995).

While it is not easy to regard Viagra use in terms of post-human anguish in the proportions of Dr Frankenstein's Monster, it is the case that the drug has unexpected and surprising effects that challenge how we think about the relationship between sexuality and technology and that translate into challenges for technosexual citizenship. Using Viagra is not a simple triumph of bio-technology over the body. Nor is it an example of straightforward bio-medicalisation of sexual experience. Viagra use turns out to be productive of forms of sexual experience and social relations that forge new engagements with self and others. Like the notional questing avatar and the necessary reciprocal relations it implies, the Viagra cyborg is also generating technosexual citizenship.

Outwardly, Viagra is a prime example of bio-technological incursion into sexual experience. It is a form of sexuopharmacy that allows men to have or sustain erections, where previously there had been difficulties. Because Viagra is so effective, it has the effect of erasing the previous explanations for erectile dysfunction, especially the psychosocial ones, such as performance anxiety and depression (Bass, 2001). Because of its effective biological action on the body, Viagra 'proves' that erectile dysfunction is biologically determined. Because Viagra has the effect of improving erections, even in situations where they were satisfactory, the drug has the effect of cutting off the sexual body from psychological and social explanations and processes. It therefore has the effect of reinforcing a bio-technological model of sexual embodiment and, by extension, the model of sexual health as the absence of disease, or in this case, erectile dysfunction. Indeed, Viagra also has the effect of displacing other explanations for erectile dysfunction such as aging (Marshall, 2002). After Viagra, there is no such medical object as an old erection. There are only more or less functional ones. According to Marshall, we now live in the age of 'erectile health'. Viagra therefore encroaches on sexuality, separating biology from psychology and social relations, rendering all sexual bodies inadequate under this new cyborg model of erections. It is argued that Viagra and similar products materialise a logic of erectile functioning derived from a masculine ideal of a perfectible, reliable penis and focused on penetrative sexual intercourse (Potts, 2005). This logic also creates a sense of inadequacy in those who do not possess such a penis (Bass, 2001). Luckily for the pharmaceutical industry, most men from time to time, can be placed in this category. Even if men do not exhibit erectile dysfunction that meets clinical criteria, the idea that a better erection is now possible is sufficient for a sense of inadequacy to arise. Or further, the possibility of an improved erection mobilises a duty to oneself to take advantage of this new technological modification of sexual masculinity. The human in this circuit of production is relegated to the role of medium through which a profitable pharmaceutical product can perpetuate itself.

As I noted in Chapter 1, Viagra has also come to feature in sexual health in a more direct way. Several studies have examined the extent to which the use of Viagra may contribute to the transmission of sexually transmitted infections, particularly HIV. A London community survey of gay men reported that one in seven had used Viagra, mostly self-prescribed (Sherr et al., 2000). These researchers also found associations between use of Viagra and behaviour that could transmit HIV. They concluded that Viagra use was a marker for risky sexual practices. Another study surveyed men attending night-clubs in Los Angeles (Fisher et al., 2006). These researchers found that Viagra use was more prevalent among gay men, but that significant numbers of heterosexual men also used it. Both groups used Viagra in combination with recreational drugs. Indeed, research has investigated the self-prescription of Viagra and illicit drugs such as methamphetamine (Halkitis & Green, 2007; Mansergh et al., 2006; Spindler et al., 2007). According to some, Viagra has entered into a culture of "... sex and drug parties" (Del Casino, 2007: 909). All this research activity serves to fix the Viagra cyborg as a sexual health concern.

However, empirical research is suggesting that the bio-medicalising effects of the Viagra cyborg are more nuanced than they appear at first glance. Employing a Deleuzian framing of embodiment, Potts and colleagues have argued that desire and bio-medicalisation do not form a straightforward relationship (Potts, 2004). This is because in a Deleuzian framework, "... desire is positive, productive, experimental and inventive, it follows no goal or direction" (2004: 20). Conversely, bio-technologisation draws on the normalising duality of pathology and abnormality. Potts and colleagues take the Deleuzian idea of "... temporary assemblages" (2004: 19) to consider, not how the Viagra cyborg comes into being, but what effects it has, or as Potts and colleagues say, 'What can a Viagra body do?'. In this light, Viagra is found to have a multitude of effects, some of which exist outside the expectations of those who use, prescribe and produce Viagra. Interviewees reported satisfaction with Viagra in the expected ways of improved erections and therefore sexual intercourse, but also reflected on the less satisfactory aspects of Viagra such as numbness and reduction in sensation or changed experience of embodiment in general. Viagra was therefore found to mobilise different forms of embodiment, sexual and otherwise. Fox and Ward have also used Deleuzian ideas to address the online prescribing of Viagra (2006). They conceptualise Viagra prescribing as a melange of orthodox prosthesis and more radical self-prescribing for pleasure. In these framings, desire is productive and radicalising of the relationship between sex and technology. These non-normative forms of sexual embodiment are in keeping with Haraway's notion of the liminal, ethical status of the human cyborg. Bio-technology can deepen reductive notions of embodiment, but it is also implicated in forms of technosexual experience that are productively disruptive.

This notion of Viagra use as productively disruptive flows into questions of medical authority over sexual embodiment. For example, in Barbara Marshall's account, Viagra is understood as a circuit of technological innovation and medicalisation (2002). As Marshall put it:

> I think that what has occurred is more the result of a sometimes uneasy and constantly shifting coalition of actors – including scientists, doctors, patients, industries, media and consumers – operating within a cultural horizon of rationalisation, medicalisation, commodification and gendered heteronormativity (2002: 146).

Marshall noted that much of the clinical research concerning sexual dysfunction is funded by pharmaceutical companies. The mobilisation of such research is thus a mix of clinical and commercial rationalities. As Marshall has pointed out, even the clinical forms of the prescribing of Viagra undermine medical authority. For fairly obvious reasons, erectile dysfunction is necessarily diagnosed by 'self-assessment', even in consultation with a doctor. The dysfunctional erection is itself rarely an object of scrutiny in clinical consultations. This practice means that the private domain of sexuality helps form a relationship between the self-determining patient-as-consumer and the research, production and sale of treatments for erectile dysfunction. Importantly, this new biotechnological relationship somewhat bypasses clinical authority over sexual functioning.

Marshall has also considered the practice of internet-based self prescription in connection with this new configuration of medical authority and sexual embodiment. Internet-based self-prescription involves purchasing Viagra and similar products via the internet. As Fox and Ward have noted, some websites that provide access to Viagra and similar products allow users to self-diagnose their sexual dysfunction and therefore assess their own suitability for sexuopharmacy (2006). *Viagra.com* is a central example. Such practices suggest how the internet facilitates forms of sexuopharmacy that deflect clinical authority. However, according to Marshall, internet-based self-prescribing only extends, or hyper-technologises, an *a priori* configuration of patient-doctor-producer concerning Viagra that already features self-diagnosis. Marshall argued that this reconfiguring of medical authority and its relation to the internet is something of a duality. It leads to a distortion and possible collapse of medical authority in the area of sexuality. But it also contributes to the 'un-mooring' (Marshall, 2002: 144) and circulation of bio-technologised notions of sexual embodiment, ready-made for corporate profit. The existence of internet-mediated self-prescription also underlines how internet and bio-technologies can be hybridised in technosexuality.

Technosexual citizenship as relational ethics

The previous sections have revealed technosexuality to be a domain for the anxieties and concerns of reflexively made online selves, the relationship between offline and online life, and struggles with the practical challenges of sustaining an ethics of online sociality. In this regard the figurative questing avatar was a central mode of online social interaction. On the basis of the questing avatar, I have made the argument that technosexuality is already ethical because reciprocity and authenticity were necessary to the ontological security of the self and therefore the effectiveness of online social relations. Via the notion of the Viagra cyborg, I made the point that technosexuality is also productively disruptive. New forms of sexual embodiment and engagements with medical authority are coming into being through the reflexive application of sexuopharmacy to sexual bodies. The Viagra cyborg lends new uses to internet-mediated communication, which in turn extends sexuopharmacy. Online sexual practice and Viagra converge in an obvious way through internet-mediated reflexivity. But there is a more foundational connection. The questing avatar and the Viagra cyborg can be regarded as particular intensifications of technosexuality joined through the general notion of self-animation mediated by technology. Seemingly quite different, they both further forms of self manipulation: one through the presentation of online selves, the ethical regulation of online intimate and sexual life, and the implications of such labour for self-awareness, identity and citizenship; and the other through the application of sexuopharmacy to the body with implications for the place of technosexual life and technosexual citizens in the bio-technology economy and systems of medical authority. In this view, technosexuality in general emerges as deeply relational. The question, How shall I be technosexual? becomes, How shall I relate technosexually? In a more abstract sense, we could also ask, What kinds of sexual relations are produced through technosexuality? This question is also foundational to public health governance of technosexuality, which strives to influence and modify the relational practices of individuals in light of the imperative of the control of sexually transmitted infections and HIV. As I noted in Chapter 1, citizenship discourse has connotations of the sovereign self and social obligation, for example, voting rights and civic duty (Giddens, 1992). In this section, I want to consider how the relational dimension of technosexuality articulates with citizenship understood in terms of the sovereign self and social obligation. With reference to research and debate concerning citizenship and sexuality and also research concerning sexually transmitted infections and HIV, I want to develop this account of technosexual citizenship as relational ethics and consider the implications for public health governance.

One theme in this discussion so far has been how technosexuality articulates with norms, expectations and imperatives. Examples included heteronormative understandings of sexual desire that inform some online sexual practices and the challenge to normative sexual embodiment that arises in relation to Viagra use. Technosexual citizenship can therefore be said to concern a general problem of reconciling the reflexive self with normativity. This problem of reconciliation makes a point of connection between technosexual citizenship and public health. In essence, public health is concerned with reconciling social actors with imperatives regarding health and illness (Petersen & Lupton, 1996). A case in point is the way public health addresses technosexuality as a potential risk for sexually transmitted infections and HIV. Often such reconciliation of self and society in terms of public health is conducted through a discourse of rights and responsibilities. For example the World Health Organisation definition of sexual health hinges on: "... the right of men and women" to sexual health (WHO, 2006: 4). This approach can lead to an opposition of the autonomous self and the social good, a conceptual framework that locks public health governance into a polarising politics for technosexuality and beyond. For present purposes, I want to make reference to three drawbacks in this framing of social action. Citizenship understood as rights and responsibilities can work to support heteronormative domesticity with implications for technosexuality. Rights and responsibility discourse does not in and of itself address social difference and therefore does not furnish methods for effectively addressing the negative aspects of technosexuality. Simple notions of citizenship have also been taken into cultural pessimism regarding sexuality (Weeks, 2007). Technosexuality is often regarded as exemplary of such pessimism, a tendency that needs to be questioned. In addition, research regarding sexually transmitted infections and HIV has revealed that rights and responsibility discourses polarise sexual subjects into model and errant citizens, with implications for public health governance.

There is a line of argument that citizenship discourse in the area of sexuality and intimate life can collapse into heteronormative domesticity. Recent legislative changes, including civil partnerships for lesbians and gay men are taken as prime examples. Diane Richardson is critical of some forms of sexual citizenship studies, typifying them as 'assimilationist', particularly those that uncritically welcome lesbian and gay marriages or civil partnership (2004). Of course, the law and sexual citizenship have a long-standing relationship. As Weeks has noted, the 1950s Wolfenden Committee inquiry and the consequent decriminalisation of homosexuality between consenting adults was an important step towards freedom for homosexually-interested people (2007). However, Weeks has also pointed out that the legislation also included clearer definitions of sex in public as crime, which meant that, in effect, many more homosexually-active men were prosecuted than ever before. Derek McGhee argued that this dynamic has continued into more recent legislative changes that have occurred in the United Kingdom in relation to sex offences against the person (2004). He noted that references to homosexuality in particular have been removed from legislation, but that there has been a concomitant generalisation of requirements on sexual conduct in the public sphere. Homosexuality is no longer the deviant other that stabilises the governance of sexuality and ensures the privileged status of heterosexuality. Instead, a more flexible approach to sexual identity is joined with a, possibly pernicious, notion of good domestic sex counterposed with bad public sex made more easily punishable under the law. Late modern sexual liberalism is egalitarian in terms of identities, but intensifies the moral ordering of sexual relating in general. As McGhee has pointed out, not all sex is 'domestic' and cautions that, in general, liberal democracies are trading freedoms for privileges in the sexual domain and in general incorporating sexualities into a kind of adapted heteronormative notion of acceptable and domesticated sexual conduct. Also addressing the law and sexuality, Cossman argued for a form of sexual citizenship that is inclusive of public forms of sexual practice and that challenges heteronormative domesticity (2002). Technosexuality is such an example. Like the internet in general, technosexuality exists in both the public and the private sphere. For example, e-dating profile postings are public, at least to other subscribers, but also intensely private in the sense that they reveal desires. It could be argued therefore that technosexuality creates special problems for the governance of sexuality, because it is not easily incorporated into heteronormative domesticity, or may work to disrupt it. Indeed, in its pursuit of technosexuality as a danger to sexual health, it does appear that public health risks aligning itself with a more general project of furthering heteronormative domesticity.

A related perspective is the homogenisation of sexual culture through its incorporation into systems of late modern capitalism. The example of the way in which Calvin Klein has sought to both trademark and produce technosexuality is a prime example, although I have argued both for the co-option of technosexuality to the logic of capitalism but also the productive potential of such consumer identities. However, Bell and Binnie have discussed what they refer to as 'gay Disneyland' (Bell & Binnie, 2004). According to these authors, as gay urban sexual spaces have become attached to local government planning for urban regeneration, they are put to the work of producing 'respectable' homosexuals and excluding undesirables. Similarly, Attwood cautioned that the sexualisation of popular culture might not reflect more openness and democratisation, but comprise a method for the expansion of the regulation of consumers through their sexuality (2006). Attwood pointed to the strongly classed and raced discourse of women's sexuality exhibited in popular television such as *Sex in the City* and *Desperate Housewives*. As we have seen in relation to Viagra, there is a well-developed critical literature concerning the way forms of technosexuality are thoroughly bound up in the logic of commercial activity. Attwood argued that we require a politics of sexual citizenship that is critical of the effects of commercial sexualisation.

In addition, rights and responsibilities discourse regarding technosexual citizenship may not effectively address social difference and persisting forms of coercive power. Indeed, there is an argument that such rights and responsibilities discourse enables forms of exploitation. Alison Adam has discussed citizenship concerns in relation to cyber-based sexual harassment of women, or e-stalking (2001). These examples of online sexual harassment included abusive and denigrating chatroom postings to websites, identity theft in the form of pretending to be the targeted woman in online communication and acting in a sexually discrediting manner, and invasion of privacy offline. Adam noted that the perpetrators were male individuals and groups. Adam argued that the internet industry response to this abuse has failed women. The industry response has been two-fold: to treat e-stalking as single episodes and therefore not relevant to overall internet use policy; or, to create universal codes of conduct that focus on 'self-protection' on the part of women users of internet services, that is, 'user beware'. Such approaches rely on a simple notion of rights and responsibilities of internet users. Adam argued that such approaches to internet ethics permit continued sexism and abuse. In particular the universal ethical strategy of responsible self-protection, expressed as the 'buyer beware' rationality of mercantilism, conflates too easily with the discourse of 'she brought it on herself' or blaming of the user in general. Adam argued for an 'ethic of care' as a way of addressing concerns such as e-stalking and harassment. By this, Adam meant that there needs to be more attention given to practices and policies that enable individuals to take action to minimise and avoid such difficulties. Adam further noted that one of the key lessons derived from the accounts of those who have had to deal with e-stalking is the informal support and assistance provided by friends and other allies found online and offline. In addition, Adam argued that it is necessary to interrogate the political and institutional frameworks that give rise to, and permit, e-stalking, including the simple notion of rights and responsibilities that appears to enable forms of exploitation.

A similar argument concerning rights and responsibilities arises in relation to biological citizenship. It has been argued that the contraceptive Pill is a bio-technology that extends neo-liberal subjectivity (Granzow, 2007). In this line of argument, the choice to use the Pill is fictive and simply another dimension of requirements on self-governing, prudent, neo-liberal subjects. However, other perspectives have been articulated. Novas and Rose have discussed the expectation of the prudent self associated with the new genetic tests for Huntington's Chorea (2000). In this research, people found to have the gene for Huntington's Chorea valued genetic testing because they wanted to make plans for their future lives, relationships and pregnancy. Novas and Rose argued therefore that requirements on conduct need not be co-extensive with neo-liberal forms of governance. They argued for an elaboration of forms of biological citizenship that value autonomy outside of neo-liberal interests. Responsibility in this view has to do with social relations, for example, decisions concerning sexual partnering and having children.

Another feature of the debate surrounding citizenship rights and responsibilities concerns a deep cultural pessimism with regard to sexual and intimate life in late modernity (Weeks, 2007). This cultural pessimism has special relevance for technosexual forms such as e-dating and Viagra use, which are often regarded as indicators of increasing promiscuity, the erosion of intimacy and family life, and the pursuit of sexual pleasure above all else. A challenge, therefore, is finding a way of engaging with sexual ethics in a critical way, that does not reinforce, or become subject to, cultural pessimism. Plummer referred to this challenge in this way:

> The idea of intimate citizenship emerges against a backdrop of debates in public spheres over appropriate ways of living life with others. In many ways it seeks to foster the civilising of relations at a time when some people see only conflict, breakdown, fear, a dumbing down of society, or a general lack of civility in social life – the new barbarisms, as they have been called. At a time when collapse of values and ethics is often said to be taking place, the concept of intimate citizenship can help show the way to new moralities and a new understanding of ethics (2003: 84).

Plummer therefore recognised the need to move away from abstract, universal ethics of sexual citizenship to grounded, everyday ethics for real world circumstances. In particular he advocated a notion of "... strategic essentialism" (2003: 83). This notion concerns a negotiable standard of social justice for late modern intimate life figured around care, responsibility, respect and knowledge. Weeks has noted how cultural pessimism expresses itself in both radicalism and conservatism:

> ... the jeremiads of Left and Right which see moral decline as the hallmark of the present too readily collapse the moral economy of capitalism with the moral agency that people exercise in their close relationships, and underestimate the nature and extent of people's resistance and resilience as they struggle with the dilemmas in their everyday lives. They confront these dilemmas in ways which remain highly gendered, and which are shaped by diverse circumstances and influences, and relational practices. But the crucial point it is worth underlining again is that despite the multiplicity of social worlds and cultural patterns, the variety of relationships and different types of family, a common normative consensus does exist around the importance of the values of reciprocity, care and mutual responsibility (2007: 178).

Like Plummer, Weeks argued for a notion of minimum universals figured around "... right to life and liberty" (2007: 162) and an: "... ethics of interdependence and mutual care" (2007: 177). Giddens has argued for something similar in his articulation of: "... intimacy as democracy" (1992: 184). Weeks made the point that social conservatism and some forms of radical post-modernism form an unwitting alliance in relation to their shared pessimism regarding the sexual self in late modernity (2007). Conservatives decry the loss of moral standards and have at times pointed to sexually transmitted infections and HIV as exemplary consequences of the break down of the regulation of sexual practice. As I noted in Chapter 1, the media hype centring on bare-backing and internet infidelity are cases in point. However, some post-modernists see dangers in humanistic notions of social progress, social democracy and other articulations of the autonomous subject, seeing these as just other forms of self-subjection to new forms of normative governance. In this view, the reflexive character of technosexuality is yet another form of disciplinary rule. Heteronormative domesticity already discussed is an example. But, according to Weeks, such pessimism in the guise of radicalism ends up collapsing autonomy with neo-liberalism. Weeks provided a picture of a broadly democratic sexuality and gender movement over the course of the 20th century and into the 21st. He argued that the autonomy that has been achieved in and around intimate life does not necessarily express an atomisation of social actors and therefore an accommodation of market-place or neo-liberal rational-ities. He further argued that regard for others is not necessarily inconsis-tent with such autonomous action. On the contrary, forms of social existence, and especially aspects of sexuality, cannot exist without some arrangement of joint action. Autonomy does not mean repudiating care of the self or of the other. Plummer and Weeks have both argued for social complexity being negotiated gradually, but inexorably, in a more hopeful direction. As I have noted, the notion derived from Novas and Rose that the responsibilities of biological citizens may exceed the inter-ests of neo-liberalism is another way of approaching this problem. Plummer and Weeks have not pretended that there are no problems. They have referred to sexual health, HIV and technosexuality, among others, as sources of challenges. Weeks also argued that same sex mar-riage is a positive step of recognition, and not as some theorists assert, necessarily self-subjection to hetero-normative expectations of intimate life. Weeks tentatively explored the extent to which the social institu-tion of marriage is itself changed by the existence of same sex marriage. In this sense, same sex marriage may be productively disruptive.

Qualitative research regarding sexually transmitted infections and HIV also lends support to technosexual citizenship as relational ethics. Corinne Squire has written about the "... insistent and instructive par-ticularity" of accounts of HIV citizenship (1999: 132). Drawing on Weeks and Plummer and other writers, Squire has made connections between citizenship and narrative in the interpretation of the stories of people living with HIV in the United Kingdom. Squire argued that "neighbour-liness" (1999: 115) was more apt than citizenship, as the former captured the qualities of shared historical, health, and interpersonal location, while the latter was too resonant with abstract notions of politics and the state. Neighbourliness also provided a useful way of bracketing together how people with HIV found ways of caring for themselves and each other. Such stories were said to perform: "... a pragmatic, contin-gent citizenship of equivalence rather than identity" (Squire, 1999: 129). Squire therefore offered a revision of the idea of citizenship that points to, not its power of constituting identity, but its relationality. Joanne Bryant interviewed heterosexual women in relation to their experiences of sexual intercourse (2006). Bryant found that interviewees did refer to notions of the thin universalism and self-determination consonant with sexual citizenship. But Bryant also noted how citizenship discourse can be turned to reinforce male privileges in sexual relations. For example, the concept of right to sexual pleasure for women could be articulated in ways that emulated how men are understood to define sexual pleasure. In this way, vaginal penetration became a central concept in the mean-ing of pleasure, diminishing other forms, and potentially reinforcing masculine notions of sexual pleasure. However, women wanted to be active in the negotiation of sexual pleasure in terms of determining the kinds of sex that happened, the right to enjoy sex, reciprocal sexual pleasuring, and questioning the assumptions inherent in genital sex and how it can be used to privilege the sexual pleasure of men. Bryant developed the concept of "... differentiated universalism" as a way of reflecting on how sexual citizenship could actually work in heterosexual relations (Bryant, 2006: 283). In this framing of sexual citizenship, dialogue regarding sexual pleasure takes central place.

Michael Brown has addressed the citizenship perspective as part of what he calls a critical geography of the moral panic concerning increases in HIV transmission among gay men in Seattle in the early 2000s (2006). Brown's work concerned what was seen as the weakening of resolve among gay men to practice safer sex. In this case, gay men reported to not practice safer sex were seen as errant citizens, turning their backs on the requirement of avoiding HIV transmission. The panic over risky sex was therefore articulated through a notion of sexual citizenship as a simple framework of the rights and responsibilities of the sovereign subject. Based on a narrative analysis of news and other texts and draw-ing on feminist literature, Brown argued that a sexual ethics that focuses on rights/responsibilities inevitably leads into a polarising discourse of model and errant citizenship. Based on a reappraisal of the epidemiology of HIV transmission in Seattle, Brown showed that the predicted general increase in HIV transmission did not transpire. Drawing on feminist notions of ethical relationality, Brown observed that obligations to others were "... inevitably contested, open and plural" (Brown, 2006: 880). On this basis, Brown argued for a relational ethics for sexual citizenship, that resembles the dialogical perspectives of Squire and Bryant, for example:

> A feminist approach to political obligation and disease ecology usefully extends the concept of citizenship on its own terms. Rather than relying on a tacit consent or a moral economy between rights and obligations, it suggests we ground obligation in an ethic of care and connection, where obligations are contested and negotiated, and grounded in everyday life (Brown, 2006: 893–894).

It is possible to argue therefore that the relational view of ethics for technosexual citizenship finds support in diverse scholarship. Citizenship as rights and responsibilities is found wanting in connection with its tendency to place too much emphasis on the responsibilities and rights of the sovereign self. This relational perspective is promising because it takes social difference as its starting point. The relational perspective draws attention to the qualities of the relationships we form with each other, permitting us to look at how we relate to one another, as opposed to questions of who we are and what rights and responsibilities are attached to such identities. This perspective therefore provides a basis for questioning public health engagements with technosexuality figured around rights and responsibilities.

Conclusion

The technosexualities I have been discussing are not simply forms of commercial advertising or science fiction curiosities. The kinds of sexual practice that arise through the internet and sexuopharmacy represent new possibilities for sexual and intimate life in our late modern world. Such forms of technosexuality create questions of self. This is most obvious in relation to the figure of the questing avatar and its implied, reflexively-made, online presence, the regulation of online relationships, or implications for offline experience. But there are also deep questions of conduct for Viagra cyborgs, concerning the production of sexual embodiment for men and women at a rapidly changing intersection of sexual pleasure as consumption, medical authority over the sexual body, and the commercial interests of pharmaceutical companies. Technosexuality has emerged in this discussion as not simply implying the ethics of citizenship, but as already, and necessarily, ethical. Online sexual sociality is not possible without recourse to reciprocity and authenticity. Technosexuality also proves to be productive in the sense of helping to alter social relations concerning consumption, medical authority and commercial activity. In addition, technosexuality is productive because it also involves the mutual extension of bio- and internet technology. Bio-technologies such as Viagra are circulated via the internet. And the internet finds new value in its capacity to provide access to information regarding such technologies, the products themselves and, therefore, their effects.

A key theme in this chapter has been the relational ethics for technosexual citizenship. This perspective builds on the foundational ethics that has been identified in cyber-ethnographies concerning online sexual and intimate life. This relational ethics for technosexual citizenship makes sense also in light of debates regarding sexual citizenship in general, and on the basis of research regarding sexually transmitted infections and HIV in particular. This relational view is not put forward as a panacea. But it does potentially avoid some of the drawbacks of citizenship understood as rights and responsibilities. The relational perspective therefore helps to move us away from an opposition of autonomy and the social good, which can lead into the demonisation of groups of people or individuals. Instead, a situated, dialogical approach to the ethics of relationality is favoured, one that is sensitive to cultural concerns such as intimacy, desire, ethical sexual relations, gender power in sexual relations, and other tensions.

In the chapters to follow, I want to further develop my account of technologically-mediated forms of sexual life with reference to public health governance. In the next chapter, I consider how communication technology, such as the internet, has been implicated in various sexual health concerns, particularly HIV transmission. I will use this discussion to critically appraise some of the assumptions that underpin public health research on the subject. In the following chapter, I build on the observations regarding internet based self prescribing of Viagra, to consider how bio- and communication technologies come together in the area of HIV prevention. This chapter will therefore be used to establish the notion of hyper-technologisation and public health governance.

3
Internet-Mediated Sexual Practices

As I have previously noted, internet-mediated sexual practices can be taken to be an important aspect of technosexuality. This chapter provides a critical overview of research concerning internet-mediated partnering, or as I will refer to it for ease, e-dating. E-dating can be defined as using the internet to secure offline meetings. My focus here will be e-dating and sexual health concerns. E-dating is often conducted through websites designed for that purpose. But sexual and romantic partnering can be established and sustained through many other forms of internet-mediation, such as those possible in online games or other internet environments. As I pointed out in Chapter 1, e-dating and related practices have been the subject of epidemiological research concerning risk for sexually transmitted infections, such as HIV. In this regard, researchers have examined whether or not the relatively recent advent of e-dating has increased the risk of HIV transmission among affected groups, particularly gay men, and to a lesser extent, young people. One of the effects of the HIV epidemic in particular and the question of sexual health in general, is to mobilise a necessary engagement with assumptions regarding the biomedical model of disease, which includes an epidemiological rationality of attending to those seen to be more at risk of HIV and sexually transmitted infections, such as gay men and young people. But biomedical knowledge can also bring with it assumptions about such people, how they act, and therefore also sexuality (Hart & Wellings, 2002). I will address the prospect of such medicalisation in the chapters to follow. For present purposes however, we need to recognise that the manner in which public health has framed much of the research regarding sexual practices that involve the internet is by no means isolated from the assumptions regarding agency that derive from the biomedical model of public health. As I have discussed in

Chapter 2, e-dating is an expression of the changes with regard to sexual and intimate life in the late modern period in general, a point not often acknowledged in public health research regarding sexual health concerns.

The first section of this chapter considers the sexual health implications of e-dating and reflects on the findings of extant research. The following section draws out the underlying determinism of much of the research addressing e-dating and sexual health. A major theme of this section will be a critical appraisal of the attribution of sexual health problems to the supposed anonymity of the internet. A related concern will be the notion of the digital closet which has to do with how the internet makes forms of sexual difference, and even 'perversity', visible in such a way as to stabilise 'acceptable' sexuality. In contrast with deterministic notions of e-dating and sexual health, the section that follows considers how e-dating could be thought of as reliant on ethical relationality. The final section considers some possible challenges to such ethics of relationality based on what can be taken to be the solipsistic and narcissistic aspects of e-dating, among other concerns.

E-dating as a sexual health risk

E-dating and related internet-mediated forms of sexual interaction appear to have become popular activities in the internet age. Accordingly, research has considered whether or not e-dating increases the transmission of sexually transmitted infections and HIV. But the findings of this research are somewhat ambiguous.

There are difficulties quantifying the use of the internet in relation to sexual practice. The technologies of the internet change rapidly and the content is itself diverse and dynamic. As I have noted in Chapter 1, Arvidsson has observed that the largest e-dating websites, *Match.Com* and *Lavalife.com*, have international operations with subscribers and revenue numbering in millions (2006). Although it is debatable that internet content is a measure of consumption, we can observe that there is a profusion of e-dating websites. A Google search of 'online dating' on the 18 January 2008 provided nearly 86 million hits, although not all of these were functioning websites. Titles found in this way included; *Bemygal.com; Christian dating for free; matchmaker.com; eharmony.com; RSVP.com.au*. According to its co-founder, *Gay.com* (accessed 10 August 2008), a US-based gay e-dating website, was so popular that at one point it was rated among the top 25 of *all websites* in terms of "… number of return visits, page views and time spent on the site ... ... [with] 10 million visits each month, with more than 100 million page views" (Ellis et al., 2002: 33).

Surveys are giving a mixed picture of the extent of e-dating, probably a reflection of how the questions are posed and if samples were drawn from an online population. For example, an internet-based survey (n=7037; 25.8 per cent reported as women) in the United States defined the sexual use of the internet broadly to include: viewing explicit images; e-dating; searching for information regarding sex; and having cyber-sex (Cooper et al., 2002). Between 9–10 per cent of both men and women reported having at some point in time used the internet for e-dating. Researchers noted that while some people did report negative aspects of such internet-related sexual activity, most did not. Another online survey of women using the internet in the United States (n=1276) reported that 43 per cent had found a partner for sex through the internet (McFarlane et al., 2004).

Offline samples add other perspectives. As I noted in Chapter 1, a survey of university students in Canada (n=760) showed that half had used the internet to seek information regarding sexual health and that such behaviour was associated with other forms of internet-based sexuality, including e-dating (Boies, 2002). Researchers have argued for the growing importance of the internet as a source of sex partners among 18–24 year old men and women (McFarlane et al., 2002). A survey of patients attending a sexually transmitted infections clinic in Denver, United States argued that gay men are most likely to use the internet for sexual purposes, but that heterosexual people use it also, albeit in smaller numbers (Rietmeijer et al., 2003). Community and online surveys of gay men in the United Kingdom between 1999 and 2001 show that the proportion who agree that they had used the internet for any reason (email, chatrooms, discussion forums) grew from 48 per cent in 1997 to 66 per cent in 2001 (Weatherburn et al., 2003). Over this period, e-dating came to be ranked as one of the most popular methods of finding new sexual partners, along with pubs and clubs.

However, the evidence that e-dating adds to sexual health risks is not overly convincing. It also seems likely that e-dating practices are subject to sexual identity and cultural expectations regarding sexual relating, somewhat questioning the view that internet technology itself contributes to sexual health risks. An online survey of women in the United States who had met an e-dating partner (n=568) showed that while women used strategies to vet their partners, a large proportion did not use condoms for penetrative sex with these partners (Padgett, 2007). This research also reported a non-significant trend where women were less likely to use condoms with their internet partners, compared with their non-internet partners. Although this finding is a trend only, it was suggested that it reflected the deeper intimacy felt for internet partners as opposed to non-internet partners. Such research needs corroboration. In addition, it might be a mistake to conclude that e-dating causes risky sexual practice, at least for gay men. For example, as Jonathan Elford and colleagues have argued, if e-dating produced risky sexual behaviour (for whatever reason), we would expect e-daters to show more risky behaviour with their internet partners compared with their non-internet partners (2006). But this does not appear to be the case. Elford and colleagues have found that gay men e-daters are no more likely to have risky sex with their internet partners (2006). Elford and colleagues did however find that gay men with HIV appeared to use the internet to find partners who also had HIV and did not use condoms. While this practice is not a risk for the transmission of new HIV infections, it may be for sexually transmitted infections. A content analysis of online dating advertisements of gay and heterosexual men showed that gay men's advertisements were twice as likely to reveal statements and requirements concerning safer sex, sexually transmitted infections and HIV (Phua et al., 2002). This finding was taken to suggest a heightened awareness of sexual health among gay men, or that heterosexual men largely ignore sexual health. Other researchers have argued that some gay men use their e-dating profiles and online messages to reveal their sexual preferences, their HIV serostatus and their approaches to HIV prevention (Carballo-Dieguez & Bauermeister, 2004; Davis et al., 2006c; Dawson et al., 2007).

Techno-determinism and cyber-perversity

While somewhat ambiguous in terms of the picture it provides, much of the research concerning the relationship between e-dating and sexual health relies on an assumption that there is something particular to the sexual partnering produced through the internet that increases risky sex. This assumption itself draws, explicitly or not, on an assumption that technologies determine society. The most obvious expression of such assumptions can be seen in research that regards the over-use of the internet for sexual purposes as a 'drug of choice' (Delmonico et al., 2002). A contrast would be research that has described a website used by gay men who like to cottage (Ashford, 2006). The point of this cottaging example its that it demonstrates not how the internet impacts on sexual practice, but how the internet mediates and contributes to its expression. While there are several forms of techno-determinism in public health research regarding technosexuality, by far the most significant of these is the idea that the anonymity of internet-based communication endangers healthy sexuality. The possibility of anonymous sexual agents is discomforting for public health wedded to forms of risk reduction that hinge on the proper arrangement of identities that serve the control of sexual health and HIV. I want to argue for something quite different. Based on the cyber-ethnographies I have already discussed which foreground the relational ethics of reciprocity and authenticity, and some other sources I will introduce here, I want to argue for 'strategic visibility'. Further I want to say that the focus on anonymity, is one part of an interest in the visibility of technosexual citizens. The notion of anonymity also mobilises a contestation of what will count as acceptable sexual practice articulated with the internet.

There are several ways in which a determinist view of technosexuality and sexual health is expressed. There is an agnostic position reflected in research that assiduously avoids referring to explanations as such, but uses statistical methods to test for associations between e-dating and sexual behaviour that may lead to the transmission of HIV and other sexually transmissible diseases. Such research treats e-dating as an independent variable in association with measures of risky behaviour. This research does provide important information regarding measures of association. But while this research avoids explanations as such, it nevertheless does not interrogate or deny them. In a sense this agnostic position permits the circulation of the other deterministic, and sometimes moralising, explanations. Compulsion is another prominent explanatory theme. Drawing on an addiction model, researchers have argued that e-dating and related practices are associated with a pattern of behaviours referred to as sexual compulsivity (Parsons et al., 2002). While a pattern of compulsive use of e-dating might be a problem for some people, it cannot on its own be an explanation or basis for sexual health interventions. Perhaps the most famous internet practice associated with risky sex is 'barebacking'. As I have discussed, barebacking refers to 'intentionally' engaging in sexual intercourse that may transmit HIV and therefore apparently acting against public health advice (Mansergh et al., 2002). Barebacking discourse is moral panic and therefore not an explanation of behaviour as such. As I will argue in the following chapters, barebacking discourse, in its most idealised formation, is risk for risk's sake. It is its own proof and in effect requires no explanation. Barebacking discourse therefore supplies a form of explanation where no other satisfactory social science one is available. In so doing, it also permits the circulation of deterministic assumptions.

However, the most significant techno-determinism regarding internet-based sexuality concerns its apparent anonymity. In a discussion of the ethical considerations that arise in forms of internet-mediated sexuality, Plummer has noted how concerns hinge around the apparent anonymity of online presence (2003: 11). Anonymity and its cousin, deception, often figure in accounts of online sexuality in general (Ben-Ze'ev, 2004). Some researchers have speculated that the internet may increase risk because e-dating provides for anonymity, although they do not discuss the precise mechanism whereby anonymity would produce unsafe sex. Researchers have developed a survey scale for measuring 'lying on the internet' (Ross et al., 2006). These researchers have tried to quantify the extent to which people themselves distort facts about themselves online and also the extent to which they believed they were being lied to. According to these researchers, age and physical attributes were common sources of distortion. Importantly, HIV status was the least distorted fact of all. These researchers also found that there were no differences in the extent of lying between online and real life. Despite ambiguities, this example underlines how questions of truth and falsehood have become central in the public health governance of internet-based sexual partnering. Indeed, one author has gone so far as to attribute the sexual effects of the internet to what is called the 'triple A engine': access, anonymity and affordability (Cooper & Griffin-Shelley, 2002). This is a clearly deterministic model of internet-based sexual behaviour. It likens the social aspects of identity management with both communications infrastructure and the economics of information technology. The central idea is that ubiquitous, cheap and above all anonymous communication drives internet-based sexual practices. There is also a psychological theory that anonymity affords social disinhibition and its internet-based manifestation, 'flaming' (Whitty & Carr, 2006: see page 67). The practice of 'flaming' refers to the situation where people engage in socially inappropriate behaviour online, such as aggression and abuse, because the norms of face-to-face interaction and social roles do not apply. As I have noted, psychoanalysts have also argued that the disinhibition thesis explains the intimacy of online life, but therefore also its psychological dangers (Young, 2002). Public health research has so far failed to explain how online disinhibition pursuant to anonymous communication translates into offline unsafe sexual behaviour. There is a kind of 'hand wavy' implication that deception or even the portrayal of a false self in some way jeopardises safer sex practices. There is also a possible contradiction in these perspectives regarding e-dating and sexual health risks. For example, Padgett argued that women were less likely to use condoms with their online partners because they had stronger feelings of intimacy for them (Padgett, 2007). Findings that lend support to the intimacy of online interaction somewhat question anonymity. Or, if we take all this research seriously and therefore combine these concepts of anonymity, disinhibition and intimacy, we are asked to encounter the rather confusing notion of 'anonymous intimacy'. While it may be possible to exercise forms of anonymous intimacy online, public health research seems somewhat inconsistent through its subscription to both anonymity and intimacy as conceptualisations of online sociality and sexual health risks. There is a further contradiction in this notion of anonymity. In abstract terms, even the making of a 'false' identity springs from imagination and desire. Falsehood is therefore already very much about identity.

In addition, the anonymity thesis sits in contrast with the cyberethnographies I reviewed in the previous chapter. These revealed that while people were strategic concerning how much of themselves they disclosed over the internet, questions of identity were deeply significant for online sociality. As Slater argued, internet-based communication has to be actively constructed and managed (Slater, 1998). For this reason, netizens shared an ethics of transparency, authenticity and ultimately social convention that provided the means for making their online communications work. As Marshall put it, internet-based communication "... disturbs the conventional borders between truth and concealment" (Marshall, 2003), meaning that the accepted ontological status of the 'true' selves of offline social life is not necessarily available to people who communicate via the internet. In his survey of online dating profiles, Arvidsson noted: "Like the Oracle of Delphi, dating profiles neither hide nor reveal: they give signs" (2006: 679).

For online social actors, identity is not necessarily pre-given, fixed, or knowable. It has to be made. Online self is therefore always becoming as a matter of reciprocal ethical relations and the technical capacities of the internet. It can be argued that anonymity is not the effect of internet-based communication, but the starting point for self-aware social actors. Such liminal, or protean selves as Turkle has written of them (1997 [1995]), are not necessarily open to forms of governance that are traditionally exercised in public health. For example, public health research relies on fixed identities such as gender, sexual preference, and disease status. This may be one reason why 'false' identity is seen as such a problem. In a sense, public health research engages with the same dilemma as do technosexual citizens, except that the challenge of making ethical online life work is taken as reason that internet-based communication could lead to risky sexual practice.

Several additional cyber-ethnographies of online sexual life bear on these questions of anonymity. On the basis of a cyber-ethnography of gay men in Japan, Mark McLelland has written of the discrepancy between 'virtual sex' and 'real sex' that he attributed to the disinhibiting qualities of online communication (2002). He argued that, because of anonymity, it appears to be easier to be sexually explicit in online communication than in the flesh, and that therefore sometimes fleshy sex does not accord with what had been imagined or planned. McLelland went on to explain that he became far more assiduous in his 'reading' of online communication as a result, which is suggestive of the need for a kind of technosexual literacy. There is an internal contradiction here however. If the expression of sexual desire online is false, how can one acquire the skills needed to properly read online communication to achieve more satisfactory offline meetings? McLelland's research suggests that the dichotomy of online as false and offline as truthful is flawed. It could be equally argued that, online communication requires its own hermeneutical skills.

Questioning the anonymity thesis more directly, Hillier and Harrison conducted research in Australia with young same sex attracted people using the internet to explore their sexualities (2007). Hillier and Harrison point out that safer spaces for young people in general are fast disappearing in our late modern urban environments. Social networking environments such as *Facebook* and *MySpace* appear to be valued by young people precisely because they provide the basis for a social life that is not otherwise possible. Drawing on Turkle's psychoanalytic notion of transitional cyberspace, the authors made an argument that developing an online presence as a gay or lesbian person is extremely important for otherwise isolated and unsupported young people. This is a space in a psychological sense of experimentation and experience for the self-identity of the user. Young people can try out a homosexual identity, gradually acquiring knowledge and skills that can be incorporated into self-identity and that can be useful in offline social environments. For young gay and lesbian people the internet provides an important method for overcoming homophobia. The informants in Hillier and Harrison's study also referred to a shared ethic of 'playfulness', that also appears to be an aspect of cyber-spaces such as *MySpace*,

Facebook and *YouTube*, and that further resonates with psychoanalytic notions of transitional space and play. The research paints a picture of emergent cyber-practices where young same sex attracted people can find affirmation for their nascent sexual identities. A similar argument has been made in research regarding coming out online among young gay men in the United States (Thomas et al., 2007).

However, Hillier and Harrison also show that young gay and lesbian users of these internet spaces appeared to value the way in which they could be anonymous in their communications, carefully exploring gay and lesbian cyber communities without jeopardising their privacy. This perspective does appear to support the notion that internet-based communication is attractive because it affords anonymity. This is the assumption that drives research that implies that the portrayal of a false self in some way or another leads to sexual health risks. However, Hillier and Harrison's research points to a major reversal of the anonymity hypothesis. In practice, young gay and lesbian people can adopt online personae that were *more* consistent with how they felt about their sexuality. Conversely, many were actually not able to be 'themselves' in offline spaces such as at school and home. In this sense and in crude terms, for these young people, internet-based identity is closer to a 'true' self than offline social interaction. This perspective destabilises the notion of anonymity and through it the truth of the self, pointing out the situatedness of all negotiations of identity and demolishing the simplistic dichotomy of offline truths and online deceptions. Hillier and Harrison also note that young homosexuals do not typically receive relevant sex education at home or at school. However, the internet does provide access to such information.

This critique of the anonymity thesis available in the work of Hillier and Harrison leads us to questions of the how internet-based sexuality articulates with heteronormativity. Addressing this issue, David Phillips has argued for a notion of the 'digital closet' (2002). For him it is mistaken to assume that in strict terms it is possible to be anonymous in internet-based communication. Aspects of the technologies that drive the internet make it possible to eventually identify any user. For Phillips, the internet is truly panoptic and anonymity is therefore fictitious. But he also argued that it is precisely the capacity of the internet to reveal the individual that forces people, in some circumstances, to seek to mask their identities. He used the example of a middle-class professional gay man managing his work- and sexually-related uses of the internet on the laptop supplied by his employer so that these practices did not cross-over and jeopardise his professional status. Phillips argued that such practices manage the panoptic aspect of the internet in a strategic way, but they also work to make sexual difference less visible in the offline world and therefore deepen forms of marginalisation. In this way, internet-mediated sexuality is figured as a kind of cyber-ghetto. However, it may not be the case that the cyber-ghetto is internally singular. Dowsett and colleagues have argued that forms of e-dating work against ghettoisation in the sense that they make it possible to recognise sexual desires "... beyond gay community" (2008: 130). Pryce has made a similar argument in connection with homosexually-interested, heterosexual men (2008). On this basis we could argue that heteronormative domesticity may be disrupted by forms of technosexuality.

It seems therefore possible to argue that the internet is respite from homophobia, and helps to reinscribe, but also potentially disrupt, heteronormativity. These perspectives imply that the notion of anonymity has ideological properties. The idea that online anonymity is associated with problematic sexual practices reinforces the idea that offline sex is acceptable and online sex is not. This ordering of sexual practices resembles the debate in sexual citizenship regarding the assimilation and domestication of sexual practices (McGhee, 2004). But in addition, heteronormativity compels some people to exploit internet-based anonymity, or as I would prefer to say, strategic visibility, to explore and establish sexual identity and practices.

It also appears that prejudice of other kinds also figure in this contestation of online sexual life. In research colleagues and I conducted concerning e-dating and sexual health among gay men in London, we argued that e-dating mediates sexual practice and therefore sexual health, and began to consider e-dating as an articulation of the social justice model of sexual health (Davis et al., 2006b; Davis et al., 2006c). This research described the e-dating practices of gay men, for example how they used websites to advertise and browse for sexual partners. Some e-daters reflexively applied the different communications media supplied by e-dating sites to signal their approaches to safer sex. In this regard, HIV antibody serostatus was shown to have importance. In particular, some gay men with HIV chose to reveal their HIV antibody serostatus in their profiles or in other aspects of online communication. The interviewees reported that doing so reduced the effects of social rejection related to HIV positive serostatus. As one interviewee reported, prejudice directed towards gay men with HIV was quite possible in e-dating environments:

... you get people that come into a room and harass people 'cos they've got HIV. You get a lot of that. Even the ordinary chatrooms like in the London chatroom you'll get, you know, there's a couple of people who are obviously disturbed ... ... you get messages come up in the main chatroom, not personal to you, but they'll say "fuck off you AIDS cunts" and all this sort of thing or "this person's got AIDS" or "'keep away from him" and things like this, you get all of that sort of thing there so you put yourself up for that when you go in there ... ... some people just look at the pictures and say "oh you look a bit thin in the face" then as far as they're concerned you know you've got AIDS and that's it. But you know, yeah I was really harassed a lot last year by this particular guy and every time I went into a chat room he would start on me ... (Davis et al., 2006c: 168).

For this reason among others, e-daters constructed their profiles and online communication to reduce such negative experiences. In this example, the interviewee indicated that he used his profile to signal his HIV serostatus:

... it clearly says on my profile that I am so it cuts out the wankers ... ... the ones that chat for hours then when they find out you are poz they 'go away' never to be seen again (Davis et al., 2006b: 466).

Such uses of the online profile technology effectively pre-empt the prejudice of others, excluding or at least minimising such interactions in the online world. We therefore argued that this practice was a way for gay men with HIV to moderate prejudice and discrimination. Overcoming prejudice is one of the premises for e-dating websites run for people with HIV (see for example: *pozmatch.com* and *HIVdate.com*).

E-dating as reflexive practice

The notion of strategic visibility in e-dating sits in contrast with notions of compulsion, moral failure and in particular, anonymity. The emphasis for critical inquiry therefore becomes not what the internet does to sexual practice and sexual health, but how e-daters exploit the technology in the exercise of their sexual practice and health care. In this view, e-dating can be taken to be a reflexive practice in the sense that e-daters self-consciously construct themselves through web environments, and, through their interactions with others, contribute to the production of techno-sexuality. A related question pertains to how such practices are enabled, exploited and constrained, and in particular, how they afford resistance of forms of discrimination to do with sexuality and HIV, or work to produce cyber-ghettoes. In this section, I will further develop these perspectives by describing and reflecting on e-dating in more detail.

It can be argued that e-dating draws some of its organising logic from personal advertising (or 'lonely hearts' columns), carried in newspapers and magazines. Arvidsson noted that personal newspaper advertisements appeared in some countries in the 1880s to help migrants find partners (2006). Print media have attempted to hold on to the market in personal advertising by combining printed advertisements and online dating services. *The Guardian* newspaper in the UK runs just such a service (*dating.guardian.co.uk/s/* accessed 10 August 2008). In this regard, personal advertisements in newspapers, e-dating and their hybrids reveal the underlying nexus of sexuality, mediation technologies and economic activity.

E-dating, as exhibited in built-for-purpose websites, has several general features. E-daters pay a subscription to an online service. For this payment, e-daters are able to upload a 'personal profile' that can be browsed by other site users. The profile will generally contain a description of the appearance of the e-dater including their age, the shape of their body and distinguishing features, their social background, work and leisure interests. The e-dater may also be able to specify who it is they would like to meet, sometimes with as much detail as they have described themselves. E-daters may also be able to upload images of themselves. Some e-dating services may permit explicit content including preferences for sexual practices and images of the e-dater naked or dressed in fetish or erotic garb. Websites with explicit content include some for people with a specific fetish, such as sadomasochism. Such websites take precautions such as 'approving' explicit content. They also protect themselves by asking users to indicate they have reached the age of consent and otherwise agree that they are not breaking any laws that pertain to them.

In addition to uploading their own profile, e-daters can peruse those of others. Websites may provide search engines that can be used on ad hoc and automated bases. As e-daters browse profiles they can leave electronic traces or messages to indicate their interest in a profile. Other e-daters can therefore approach those who have expressed interest, or ignore them. In this regard, e-dating is reminiscent of SMS text messaging (and its precursor, the telephone answering machine). One of the men I interviewed in research concerning e-dating and HIV prevention, put it this way:

Well it's there for people to make choices. I'm gonna look at people who have sent me messages. I'll send people messages. If I'm not interested, I'll say: "No. Sorry. Thanks for the message, but not what I'm looking for". I'll always say something polite. (Davis et al., 2006b: 465)

E-dating therefore is seen to permit actors to manage their social interaction in an efficient manner. Reciprocity and a kind of minimal courtesy are also expected.

Other features of e-dating sites are Internet Relay Chat (chat) and messaging. In these parts of such sites, e-daters can conduct synchronous or asynchronous interactions with individuals or groups of e-daters. These chats or emails can be focused on clarifying the candidate's suitability for a date and on that basis, arranging it. E-daters may also shift their interactions off-site onto alternative forms of electronic communication such as email, messaging, SMS texting, and even the 'retro' telephone.

E-daters are therefore engaged in a kind of art of online presence of the sexual self, assembling images and texts that convey their desirability and that mobilise connections with interested parties. E-dating communication appears to be 'hypertextual' in the sense that, as with the internet in general, it has no definite beginning and end and can be understood as a fluid network of texts and flows that 'evolve and mutate' (Mitra & Cohen, 1999). The internet therefore has an evanescent quality through the self conscious management of appearance and disappearance. Reproducibility, dissemination *and* impermanence characterise internet-based sociality. E-daters therefore enter themselves into fluid networks of informational and symbolic exchange that are informed by their sexual and relationship interests of e-daters. The ethics of reciprocity I noted in Chapter 2 are important in this regard. Conjointly, an internet-based, sexualised and relational sociality is gradually developed. One finds oneself in this network by ensuring that one's social and sexual appeal is managed, including making the necessary adjustments to refashion or reinvigorate network connections. E-dating also bears the time/space distanciation properties of mediated communication. E-daters can interact in real-time or not with other e-daters, locally of globally. Through these various manipulations of images and texts, e-dating brings the inscription, dissemination, consumption process of mediated communication very close together. As Mitra and Cohen have noted in relation to the internet, e-daters also have a dual role in that they are both readers and writers (1999). They can peruse webpages and other products. But they can also make their own if they choose. Elsewhere, colleagues and I have argued that synchronous chat room users are aware of their hybrid role of readers/writers (Davis et al.,

2004). In such situations, chatters become adept at forms of hyper-editing of their online communication to reduce ambiguity and otherwise ensure that the chat effectively conveys intended meanings.

Another feature of e-dating concerns how it blurs and bridges spheres of social action. For example, posting a profile concerning one's sexual preferences creates an edgy mix of intimate confessions and public representations. E-dating requires that users create a narrative of the sexual self for the consumption of other prospective e-daters. In this way, the private sphere is extended into a new kind of public domain to create a mixing of these. E-daters do have some control over what they reveal, but the general imperative is to reveal in some way one's interests and aspirations so that other e-daters can decide whether or not they will make contact. In this way my previous argument regarding the internet as a social technology of visibility is relevant. In addition, the overarching rationality of e-dating means that it bridges online and offline social interaction. E-daters use the sites to organise meetings. E-dating can also work in the reverse. Several of the gay men I interviewed reported that they had invited people they met in bars to view them online and get in touch if they liked what they saw. Because of the codification and the construction of networks, offline connections are, to some extent, systematically predetermined. Sexual and relational interests are negotiated online and therefore partially predetermine the shape and operation of offline networking. Offline sexual and relationship interaction is therefore partially pre-empted by the informational and symbolic codification and relays of online sexual networking. Belinda Smaill has made a similar point (2004). E-dating works to re-embed the local, in the sense that e-daters use the internet to meet someone in the flesh. But this is not to say that online communication absolutely determines offline meetings. Turkle has described at length how even committed online interactive game players sometimes meet each other in offline conventions and parties (Turkle, 1997 [1995]). These meetings are said to have a precarious quality because, sometimes, expectations are not met and therefore meetings can be bland or disappointing.

Another important aspect of the art of online presence is the imperative that e-daters make themselves desirable to the desired other, at least up until the point where dialogue or negotiation can occur via chat and messaging. One's entrance to online presence is an assemblage of images and texts that will hopefully provide the catalyst for imagined, desirable connections. This perspective brings into play sexual and emotional fantasy, partly explaining the erotic frisson of e-dating and other sexual uses of new media. However, because of this focus on fashioning oneself in light of the imagined desires of the desired other, the ostensibly relational practice of e-dating appears to have a pronounced solipsistic dimension that raises questions concerning narcissism. Smaill has made this argument in connection with the Australian e-dating site *RSVP.com.au* (2004). Like many researchers of the area, Smaill made a claim that anonymity is an organising principle of online communication. As I have argued, this perspective sits in contrast with other cyber-ethnographies and my own position regarding the internet as a technology of visibility. Even Smaill discussed the significance of the online publication of photographs, which does suggest that visibility is important. However, Smaill noted that the self portrayed in online communication, such as in profiles and chat, is constructed so as to further one's appeal in the eyes of the desired other. Smaill argued that: "The writing of the advertisement is, in actuality, a complex folding together of self and desired other." (2004: 97) and: "In the case of online personals, identity is formulated in a manner whereby the other takes shape as an ideal that is foundational to the projection of the self" (2004: 98). Smaill implied that the fantasies, desires and aspirations of the e-dater are revealed both in how they portray themselves, but that also, this self is a projection of the imagined expectations of the desired other. Turkle referred to online communication as a kind of "mirror" (1999: 6343). Marshall made a similar comment regarding netsex, the form of sexual interaction that involves avatars in online game environments (2003). According to him, because of the technical capacities of game environments, netsex can involve writing in the responses of the other avatar on their behalf. Marshall's example suggests that it is almost as if one can write the agency of the desired sexual other into existence. This sexual agency as ventriloquism underlines the possible narcissism of internet-mediated sexuality.

Much like Slater's account of the sex pic trade, e-dating is also revealed to be a highly regulated form of online interaction. Drawing on notions of reflexive modernisation and the pure relationship, Michael Hardy conducted interviews with heterosexual men and women using an e-dating website in the United Kingdom (2004). Hardey argued that users valued e-dating because it provided for forms of increased control over the dating experience. Hardey argued that women in particular enjoyed the ways in which e-dating helped to pre-empt how the date would proceed and provided forms of volition that were harder to exercise in the face-to-face situation. For example, e-daters used their online profiles and the ensuing online chat to help them select candidates for face-to-face encounters. Interviewees also noted how they could terminate an interaction with minimal social repercussions. If a candidate appeared to fall short of one criteria or another, e-daters reported that they need not interact with them any longer. If someone was cruel or rude, e-daters simply closed the browser window. Hardey pointed out that in offline social interaction, it is not as easy to terminate social interaction, particularly it would seem, for women in some situations. Hardey also argued that e-dating made it possible for different kinds of intimacies to emerge. For example, some women e-daters found that the men they chatted with were able to take risks with their masculinity. They did so by chatting about their feelings and desires, something that the women found both untypical of men and attractive.

Drawing on Goffman's notion of the interaction order and also Giddens's notions of trust and security, Hardey argued that several 'unwritten rules' underpinned how e-daters coordinated interaction and protected themselves from negative dating experiences. Turkle was among the first to discuss the central dilemma of e-dating concerning meeting up with someone who turns out to be different from expectations (1997 [1995]). It seems that e-daters have developed strategies for just these situations. In general, it is not possible to sustain a false self if one wants to actually meet offline. If an e-dater misrepresents their appearance or other aspects of self to secure a date, other e-daters feel that it is appropriate to terminate the in-flesh date. E-daters have also developed strategies for pre-detecting distortion and falsehood by asking direct questions in chat. E-daters are also quite aware that there is a paradoxical aspect in the expectation of truth in combination with the other expectation that e-daters put their 'best foot forward'. In the research interviews I conducted with gay men in London, I found similar rules of engagement (Davis et al., 2006b; Davis et al., 2006c). For example, e-daters used chat and messaging to 'check out' the potential date, particularly focusing on age and appearance.

This focus on regulating the bonafides of the online self supports my thesis regarding strategic visibility. As noted, some do argue that internet-based communication practices such as e-dating are attractive because of the anonymity they afford. And as I have discussed, some base their arguments concerning sexual health risks on that supposition. However, the research I have discussed can be taken to suggest that anonymity is not at all categorical in e-dating practices. Some aspects of self are in play, even if the actors are not aware of them (see Turkle's account of cyber romance and the unconscious: 1997 [1995]). It is also the case that individuals are traceable online and therefore accountable, as I have already noted. In addition, one can only hold on to anonymity as the organising principle of online communication if one also privileges offline embodied co-presence over online interaction, and therefore as somehow exhibiting a truer version of self. Others argue quite convincingly that online communication practices are attractive precisely because they bypass the social judgements common in our societies related to identity and appearance, but that the online social experience is no less real for that reason. As I have noted, Carter has written about the formation of online relations as reversing the process of offline friendship formation and intimate partnering (2005). In offline worlds, one gets to know someone from the 'outside in'. In online words, actors meet the 'person within' first. This transparent self of online dating environments fits with the other notable aspects of e-dating such as the emotional closeness that some do report they experience in their online communication (Turkle, 1997 [1995]).

The situated, interactive strategies figured around visibility are suggestive of the relational ethics of technosexuality. As I noted in Chapter 2, Adam has discussed cases of online stalking, identity theft and sexual abuse of women (2001). Adam advocates the promotion of a cyberethics of reciprocal care as a method for addressing the unbridled individualism of the commercial internet. Based on the research already discussed, it does appear that heterosexual, homosexual and other sexually interested e-daters have invented situated ethical standards and related practical communication strategies to protect themselves and support each other in their use of the internet. These rules can be explicit in the conditions of use for subscribers of particular sites. But they are also informal and to some extent invented by the e-daters themselves. In addition, these rules of engagement appear to extend to HIV prevention. One e-dater put it this way in an online chat room interview:

> <Interviewee> ... I set up a new profile that said "Never" to safe sex and I was completely blatant about my HIV status—it was only alluded to in the former profile ...
> <Interviewee> I had changed my old profile to use some of the euphemisms to allude to POZ status so I presume he did ...
> <MD> what are some of the euphemisms ...
> <Interviewee> "Positive outlook on life" ...
> <Interviewee> My uncompromising stance is less than 12 months old.
> <Interviewee> Yes.
> <MD> What uncompromising stance is that?

<Interviewee> That I only have unprotected sex.

<MD> What made u change?

<Interviewee> Realising that I much preferred it.

<MD> What made u adjust yr profile

<Interviewee> For the majority of the period since I was diagnosed I had had only protected sex.

<MD> Can u expand?

<Interviewee> Realising that every man was out for the most pleasure HE could get—why should I not have the same rule?

<MD> So is this a way for you to get pleasure while reducing HIV risk?

<Interviewee> It is also only in the last 15–18 months that I had realised there was such a large subculture of POZ men having unprotected sex.

<MD> What made u realise that?

<Interviewee> I think that the number of profiles on gaydar explicit about that has risen markedly in that period.

<MD> How do you feel about being open about yr status on the net?

<Interviewee> I think it is important (Davis et al., 2006b: 166–167)

This extract reveals an engagement with e-dating and HIV prevention. It implies the existence of an internet-mediated milieu, whose members can recognise and interpret identity labels, approaches to HIV prevention, and practices of e-dating. Practices such as these may comprise a 'cyber-community of intelligibility' or 'recognition' applied to sexual health. It also implies the technological mediation of sexual relations that conform to a particular approach to living with HIV and engaging with the imperative of avoiding the transmission of HIV. This communicative strategy reflects a way of ordering risks for HIV transmission and other sexual health concerns in connection with the exercise of sexual pleasure. But, above all, it reveals an ethics of e-dating, presentation of self and HIV prevention that valorises the online transparency of such practices. As such, this approach sits in opposition to the notion of anonymity and how it is used in some public health research I discussed in the previous section. The communicative strategy builds on the identity management strategies I have also noted, particularly those that seek to avoid or reduce prejudice. The extract is also important because it points to a provocative use of knowledge about HIV serostatus derived from HIV bio-technologies. In addition, it resembles the supposedly problematic barebacking discourse that is associated with e-dating. This mixing of internet-based communication and bio-technology is the subject of the next chapter. For present purposes it is sufficient to point out that e-dating communication is one way of engaging with bio-technological knowledge. Further, because it requires a community of intelligibility, it may be that internet-mediated communication is one method through which engagements with bio-technologies that impinge on sexual practice come into being as social practices. As I will explain in the next chapter, these self-made strategies open up HIV prevention to productive disruption, in terms of the contestation of knowledge and public health governance. As I will argue in the chapters to follow, this disruption is neither a resistance of good public health government nor a new normalisation of sexual conduct. This situation needs to be understood as necessary contestation that permits engagements with the ethical questions that arise in the use of the bio-technologies themselves.

Narcissism and other challenges

Understanding e-dating as a self-consciously produced practice goes some way in critiquing common understandings of the relationship between the internet and sexuality. However, there is a deeper tension underpinning e-dating to do with autonomy, constraint and exploitation. For example, there is a contrast between Hardey's depiction of e-dating and the cyber-feminism on the subject. Hardey argued that women enjoy the increased control over the dating experience that e-dating environments appear to furnish. However, some online websites are marketed to women on just this basis. It may be therefore that the notion of e-dating as a way of exercising power on the part of women may actually provide a way for reassuring women, and therefore encouraging them to make themselves available to men. Certainly, the cyber-feminism that has begun to interrogate online gender and sexuality politics provides a picture of exploitation and corporate indifference. In addition, the solipsistic aspects of e-dating I have noted, may work against relational ethics. In this section I want to consider some possible negative aspects of e-dating concerning exploitation and narcissism, perspectives that themselves derive from the culture industry critique that has been widely applied in the area of media studies.

Internet-mediated partnering for intimate and sexual purposes sits in tension with critical theory that has been applied to mediated communication, particularly the broadcast media, such as television. For example, the culture industry critique argues that broadcast media addresses a passive mass of individual consumers (Holmes, 2005). It is also said that broadcast media reduces the aesthetic value of culture through the industrial logic of commodification and replication. A central argument is that broadcast media send messages out to multiple recipients and therefore the symbols in circulation are constructed by the few for the consumption of the many. This perspective is the basis for arguments concerning hegemonic rule and even propaganda. The rise of the internet has required a rethink of such assumptions regarding the mediatisation of societies. E-dating, like the new interactive media in general, is dialogical in the sense that e-daters can mutually influence the symbolic exchange of messages that are circulated in the internet. It would seem that the typical critical argument regarding broadcast media does not apply to the new media. However, David Holmes has argued that, despite its interactive potential, the new media extends the homogenising and individualising properties of the broadcast media (2005). He argued against the idea that the interactive aspects of the internet make it distinct from broadcast media, because: "Most internet identities are avatars for whom reciprocity is not possible" (Holmes, 2005: 150). Holmes asserted that, because of its hypertextual and therefore fluid character, the internet does not provide the social conditions for true reciprocity. This idea jars with the perspectives provided by cyber-ethnographies I have discussed regarding necessary reciprocity. It may be however that e-dating is an exception to Holmes's thesis. It is quite possible that online sexual and romantic life requires reciprocity in ways that other forms of online communication do not.

But Holmes's perspective does help raise some possible questions regarding e-dating. To some extent the practices of online profile construction are homogenising because they ask e-daters to depict themselves according to preset criteria. For example, in e-dating websites, subscribers use criteria such as the following to describe themselves: age; height; hair and eye colour; body shape; attire; ethnicity; sexual preference, and so on. Further, partner selection is also derived from a similarly limited universe of preset criteria. This aspect of e-dating could be construed as codifying the sexual self and sexual relating to make it amenable to both the technical capacities of the website environments and profitable exploitation. This is the point made by Andil Gosine in relation to race and e-dating (2007). According to Gosine, the ethnicity categories of e-dating websites require that subscribers submit to assumptions about race built into the website environments and also exercised in the online presentations and dialogues of e-daters themselves. For example, online communication appears to build on the categorisations built into the websites that require e-daters sort themselves into 'white' and 'non-white'. Whiteness emerges as the desirable normative racial identity, around which other racial identities are articulated. Online depictions of ethnicity are also seen to draw on such racist stereotypes. Like Slater discussed in the previous chapter, Gosine noted that these practices contradict the view of the internet as a space where society is not encumbered with the social differences that structure offline life. Likewise, Dowsett and colleagues have noted that African American men using gay men's e-dating websites, attend to racism by challenging reductive racial categories (2008).

The exploitation of e-daters goes beyond ideas of race. Arvidsson has noted that *Match.com* is marketed on the basis that it provides access to so-called 'quality' men and women seeking partners (2006). Arvidsson noted that subscribers are asked to be accurate in their self presentations. The e-dater is expected to not overreach themselves and therefore to place themselves 'accurately' in a hierarchy of erotic and social value. Arvidsson made the point that e-daters are not compelled to undertake this hierarchical organisation of themselves (2006). In this sense, e-dating is not constraining, but a from of self-subjection. The racist hierarchy of e-dating sites noted by Gosine and Dowsett is a similar form of self-discipline. *Match.com* e-daters incorporate themselves into a system that commodifies their value as a matter of self-evaluation. E-daters so organised into hierarchies of 'quality', become the main selling point for the website. Arvidsson pointed out how remarkable it is that e-daters organise themselves in ways that provide the basis for the commercial success of the websites, suggesting that this logic is in fact a central operating principle for the commercial aspects of the internet in general.

The culture industry critique also argues that mass mediation caters to a narcissistic individual (Holmes, 2005). This is because capitalist social organisation is said to alienate people from each other and from themselves. This media appeal to narcissism also means that individuals replace 'authentic' social relations with the satisfaction of selfish desires, relational or otherwise. Individuals are therefore said to be primed to eagerly consume the dazzling monological address of the broadcast media. E-dating could also be said to be narcissistic. As I have noted in the section above with reference to Smaill and others, e-dating has a solipsistic turn because it requires that one projects oneself in terms of the imagined desires of the desired other. Despite the overall logic of locating partners and implied interaction, the forms of self-presentation in e-dating sites can be taken to reinforce the self-absorption of late modern social life and deepen a kind of psychosexual solipsism. In line with Marcuse, forms of internet-mediated sexuality may represent 'repressive desublimation' (1972 [1964]). According to this theoretical mix of Freud and Marx, capitalism relies on forms of repression of the sexual instinct, but also its rationed expression in ways that suit economic exploitation. Because it can be taken to express repressive desublimation in such an obvious manner, e-dating could be taken to have the proportions of a cultural joke.

Through this narcissistic hypothesis, it may also be that e-dating is anti-social. Referring to Freud, Bauman has pointed out that the capacity to live as for the other is a key form of agency for the constitution of civil society (Bauman, 2003). Civil society relies on individuals to some extent reconciling their own desires with those of others. Without this ability there would be no society. In addition, this productive tension is also implied in forms of sexual health that address the individual and how they act for the good of the other. In this light, it could be argued that e-dating inhibits this reconciliation of desires because it privileges the narcissistic self. E-dating therefore promotes essentially anti-social forms of civic life in the sexual domain, or at least, does not ordinarily provide the basis for building society because individuals are committed to creating images and texts of themselves in light of what they imagine their ideal other would desire. Additional questions arise concerning the kinds of relationships that are coming into being and disappearing. This narcissistic critique is a strong challenge to the notion of a relational ethics for technosexuality. However, it can also be argued that this critique only applies to online depictions of self that are fixed and therefore primarily monological. Online communication in chatrooms and messaging is interactive and, I would argue, negotiated. Communicating to secure a date provides less scope for narcissistic forms of a supposed anti-civil society. In addition, e-daters can adjust their online profiles after feedback from others, somewhat deflecting the idea of e-dating as total narcissism. However, there may be virtue in holding onto this narcissism critique for the purposes of theory development. E-dating could be said to exhibit a *productive* tension between the narcissistic sexual self and the social relations necessary for sexual partnering. This notion of tension is more in keeping with Turkle's account of the experience of online communication as a potential learning experience (1997 [1995]).

In addition, the culture industry critique in general implies that the internet, and quite possibly e-dating along with it, inhibits social democracy. The internet in particular was often said by utopian visionaries to be the technology that would usher in a new golden age of creative, democratic life (Mosco, 2004). However, those in the more cynical, dystopian line of argument, such as Holmes, regard the media, including the internet, as methods of ideological domination. It is said that, even the new media, as interactive as it may be, atomises selves and therefore does not provide the basis for collective organisation for social democracy. Holmes argued therefore that there is no public sphere in cyberspace where a truly democratic life can be exercised (2005). It may be therefore that e-dating is one way in which the new media stifles social democracy. Smaill (2004) has also developed a kind of culture industry argument based on the notion of the 'enterprising individual' of e-dating. For example, Smaill argued that the consumer identity politics of e-dating operates as a kind of imperative whereby failure to locate a partner becomes a personal responsibility.

It is common for e-dating websites to promote themselves in terms of the exercise of the free agency of the user. For example, *Gaydar.com* (accessed 10 August 2008), a popular gay men's e-dating website, markets itself with the slogan: 'What you want, when you want'. This slogan fuses the agency of the user, sexual desire and the promise of infinite technological capacity. The internet in general is deeply implicated in the notion of the enterprising individual. One of the most significant developments in the internet was 'browsing', where, to some extent, users became able to inspect web-pages and 'surf' according to their own preferences (Hardey, 1999). Browsing was partly developed to address a practical problem of the size and rapid growth in online knowledge that made traditional systems of knowledge access, such as indexes, unworkable. In a sense, the idea of an internet user free to browse is an assumption that reflects and has enabled the development of the internet. But this notion of free choice also fits with contemporary political rationality of consumer culture. On this basis, the promise of e-dating sites as methods for finding love, intimacy and satisfying sexual interaction is to some extent mythical. As Smaill put it: "... this particular intersection between technology and culture may be seeking the promises of intimacy, but this search is bound to the auspices of capitalist aspiration" (2004: 104). Smaill did try to retrieve e-dating by considering if there is scope for something positive in the play of such consumer identities, but her argument was not strident. The conventionality of the sexualities of the internet noted by Slater in the previous chapter, reinforce this idea of internet-mediated sexual interaction as homogenised and regulated. John Tomlinson has argued that internet-based technologies both enhance and inhibit intimacy (1999).

Tomlinson relied on Giddens's notion that processes of globalisation work to increasingly separate people from themselves and each other as their daily lives become organised around labour, consumption and parenting. In this context, part of the attraction of e-dating and internet-based communication in general, is that it promises to overcome such sequestration of everyday life, breaking down social isolation by bringing about new connections and by implication new kinds of intimacies fitted to late modern social circumstances (Tomlinson, 1999: 169). Tomlinson also suggested that as globalisation processes have altered the practice of democracy and deepened the significance of intimacy, these have found a new connection, which does support the view of the scholars of sexual citizenship such as Plummer and Weeks. But Tomlinson is sceptical of the kinds of mediations of intimacy afforded by the internet and by extension e-dating. He sees that online communication practices foster forms of "... moral detachment", among other effects (1999: 176).

It is also possible to argue that the sublimation of desire reflected in e-dating keeps the internet functioning. Desire for social and sexual connection is harnessed to the internet, in a sense that echoes the science fiction depictions of technology exploiting humans, such as in the *Matrix* films. In this line of argument, e-dating becomes a technology that seeks to perpetuate itself. There is no hegemony in play as such, save the logic of autopoiesis of e-dating itself, and therefore the internet in general (van Loon, 2008). But equally, there is little scope for democratic engagement. E-dating could be therefore construed as one means of negating the body politic. However, apart from the forms of cyberstalking identified by cyber feminist researchers, it is not clear that internet-mediated partnering should be singled out as an especially problematic distortion of social democracy. Perhaps the only important critique derived from this line of argument is that e-dating is an ideology vacuum, in terms of democracy at least, and therefore works as a kind of cultural anaesthetic. Individuals may not be necessarily dominated by a pernicious framing of politics embedded in e-dating websites, or, necessarily, an inhibition of democratic sociality. But they may well be asked to render themselves as libidinous zombies or lonely post-humans, or both.

It also needs to be recognised that the culture industry critiques themselves have has some problems. For example, all interaction, that is online and offline, is informed by a projection of self to suit the desires of the imagined other. It is a Freudian cliché, but narcissism is said to be a feature of all social life. In addition there is a kind of implicit nostalgia in a critique that assumes a pure culture that existed before mediation, and in the present case, halcyon sexual cultures before e-dating. The critique also underestimates the critical literacy of individuals themselves. As the previously discussed research serves to reveal, e-daters are thoroughly engaged with the capacities and limitations of the e-dating technologies. The idea of the homogenising of sexual cultures also sits awkwardly with the current mythology of the internet as a place where sexual desire and in particular, perversion, is exercised to the detriment of society. The culture critique does not explain very well how it is that e-dating could be exploitative by offering forms of sublimation as domination but also be transgressive and therefore a social problem.

Conclusion

E-dating provides an important case study for technosexuality and public health. The idea that e-dating in some way might cause sexual health problems is implicit or explicit in much public health research on the topic. But supporting research evidence is not strong. While e-daters do take risks, it appears that gay and other homosexually-interested men are no more likely to do so with their online partners, compared with their offline partners. We cannot be sure if the same applies to heterosexual people as there is so little research on the subject. However, it seems likely that we should not assume that internet-mediated social and sexual partnering produces sexual health risks in the deterministic sense. But equally, the practice of e-dating and the communication technologies it relies on, do create new implications for sexual health. Despite such ambiguity, much public health research and even some cyber-ethnographies persist in their reliance on the idea that the internet is problematic because it allows people to communicate anonymously. I argued that this idea of anonymous communication is an oxymoron because effective communication online requires some transparency. In addition, the question of anonymity, or more properly truthfulness, relies on an opposition of offline and online reality. The idea of anonymity in online communication presupposes that offline communication is somehow more authentic and therefore closer to the truth. This line of argument is in fact both epistemologically and ontologically problematic. For example, it is quite possible to be untruthful in the offline world. Authenticity is therefore always a potential social issue. If internet-based communication does have a systematic effect in relation to identity and social relations, it is that it destabilises our assumptions regarding offline life. Online sociality reveals the made, or even arbitrary, quality of identity and social relations in the offline world. The most salient example of the limitations of the anonymity thesis concerned the online coming out of lesbians and gay men, who found that they could be more true to themselves online than anywhere else!

It is possible to argue therefore, that anonymity is not so much an explanation of the effects of the internet in sexual life, but a method for the government of technosexuality. It provides a way of summarising the effects of the internet on communication that mandates the scrutiny of the truthfulness of online citizenship. The anonymity thesis suggests that forms of panoptic exploitation of the technical capacities of the internet are coming into being, not least of all, through public health research regarding sexual health. This notion of the internet as a method of surveillance can be brought into connection with sexual politics and specifically difference. For example, the formation of cyberghettoes and the digital closet, suggest also that the relegation of perversity to the internet works to stabilise acceptable forms of sexuality. Technosexuality may be the required other of heteronormative domesticity.

In response to this critique of the anonymity thesis, I invited the reader to consider the notion of strategic visibility. This notion helps reframe anonymity, recognises how people actually make e-dating work, and permits connections with the relational ethics of online intimate life. The research I have discussed does appear to suggest that in their online interactions, e-daters are striving to develop a situated ethics that helps to resolve all manner of dilemmas such as, the trustworthiness of the prospective partner, the moderation of social rejection, and stigma for people with HIV. However, through a discussion of the culture industry critique, I also suggested that the possibilities for a relational ethics in e-dating in particular, or technosexuality in general, is possibly compromised by the ways in which narcissism can be put to the service of the logic of profitable exploitation and the numbing of the democratic possibilities of the internet.

Another theme of this chapter that is so far underdeveloped is the relationship between e-dating and the knowledge produced by biotechnologies that have relevance for sexual health. The example I used was the e-dater who made HIV serostatus and HIV prevention intentions transparent in online communication. Examples such as these draw attention to agency in connection with bio- and communication technologies and how these practices are informed by the imperatives of public health. While, as I have suggested, causation is a problematic direction of inquiry, it can be argued that sexual health is, in part, mediated by the practice of e-dating. In the next chapter, I want to expand on this theme concerning the mixing of bio- and communication technologies in sexual practice.

4
HIV Bio-Technologies and Sexual Practice

As the previous chapter noted, internet-based communication strategies can be used to moderate negative social experiences and manage sexual health risks. In this chapter, I will take the case of HIV bio-technologies to argue for 'hyper-technologisation' or the mingling of bio- and communication technologies. Such hypertechnologisation is apparent in the area of sexuopharmacy, where internet-prescribing is said to 'un-moor' the Viagra cyborg from traditional forms of prescriber/patient relations (Marshall, 2002). As noted, Viagra itself has been considered as a possible risk factor in research regarding HIV prevention (Halkitis & Green, 2007). Here I want to argue that the relationship between bio- and communication technologies is in part forced into existence by the imperative of HIV prevention. In particular, I want to address practices such as the so-called, internet-mediated 'serosorting', which concerns the notion of using communication technologies to choose a partner of the same HIV antibody serostatus. Such notions will be used to consider how, along with communication technologies, bio-technologies help mediate sexual practices. There have been general calls for closer attention to the social aspects of technologies used in the prevention of HIV, such as using short-term treatment to prevent HIV transmission after sexual exposure (Imrie et al., 2007). Such a literature is emerging (Nodin et al., 2008). I want to contribute to this literature through an argument that much of the research applied to the question of HIV prevention and bio-technologies subscribes to a determinist view of sexual action. As such, this research is consistent with the determinism that is extensively employed in research regarding e-dating, sexually transmitted infections, and HIV. Determinism is undoubtedly attractive because it is consistent with the effects of bio-technologies in the control of HIV infection. However, such research has its own problems and does not necessarily support the deterministic view, even by its own criteria. I will take the view that it is the requirement of HIV prevention that imbues bio-technologies with implications for sexual relationships. This may seem obvious, but it is a reversal of the standard research approach, which explores the impact of bio-technologies in sexual practice and not the importance of public health rationalities for the articulation of bio-technological effects. On this basis, I want to consider the work that both bio- and communication technologies are put to inside public health governance.

Many of the examples I will draw on in this chapter concern gay and other homosexually active men in affluent countries, with access to the full and emerging range of HIV bio-technologies. However, the argument I want to make here is likely to be relevant for other groups and places. In particular, the logic of serosorting derived from the HIV antibody test is implied in the example of the Safe Sex Passport, which, as I have discussed, addressed any sexually interested online citizen, at least in the United States. The logic of the passport relied on tests for sexually transmitted infections and HIV, which are widely available. I am therefore proposing that, although there may be local and identity-linked variations, hypertechnologisation has relevance for the public health governance of sexually transmitted infections and HIV in general.

At the outset of this discussion, I want to be clear that I am not trying to argue that hyper-technologisation determines sexual relations. For example, what people say and do online may not be completely coherent with what happens in offline sexual situations. Such lines of causation are difficult to establish in any research. In addition, it is also possible that people who identify themselves as HIV negative but suspect they are HIV positive (because they have not recently tested) may not behave as do people who say and know they are HIV negative. Such subtleties are yet to be thoroughly researched. My objective is therefore modest. I want to show that public health does not stand outside technosexuality, but is actively involved in its production, and in particular, works to join bio- and communication technologies.

In the sections that follow, I will first explain the significance of bio-technology for HIV prevention. I will do this with reference to the advent of effective HIV treatment and by providing some information regarding bio-technologies that support it. I will then turn to the research that has addressed the relationship between sexual practice and knowledge regarding HIV transmission derived from HIV bio-technologies. I will identify what such research suggests regarding how public health is implicated in hyper-technologisation. In the final section, I will discuss how HIV bio-technologies and their hybrids with communication technologies have been incorporated into sexual cultures.

The advent of effective HIV treatment

HIV treatment is a paradox for public health governance. Improvements in the control of HIV infection have led to concerns of a post-treatment epidemic. These concerns take several forms. Some have argued that, because of treatment, people now no longer fear HIV/AIDS so practice safer sex less often. Others have argued that knowledge that HIV treatment inhibits the action of the virus is leading people to practice safer sex less often. Practitioners have also become concerned that drug-resistant forms of HIV are developing and, through 'reinfection' of people with HIV, are leading to an untreatable HIV epidemic (Salomon et al., 2000). Accordingly, research has concerned itself with the risk of increased spread of HIV related to aspects of HIV bio-technologies (Elford, 2006). Policy makers and researchers have also called for interventions to increase altruistic conduct on the part of people with HIV regarding HIV prevention in efforts to halt the post-treatment spread of HIV (Janssen et al., 2001). These assumptions imply that treatment influences sexual and HIV prevention practice in much the same way as it influences viral activity. For example, the history of HIV treatment is often understood in terms of a technologically-determined watershed. The Vancouver World AIDS Conference in 1996 has been referred to as this watershed moment (Holzemer, 1997). At this conference, research was announced that confirmed the efficacy of HIV treatment. This watershed assumption assumes that the history of the epidemic is singular and that the advent of effective HIV treatment has altered the course of that history. It is not my interest to deny that HIV treatment is effective (for a description of the reduction in death and morbidity since the introduction of effective HIV treatments, see: *aidsmap.com/ cms1032117.asp* accessed 10 August 2008). But I am interested to distinguish between such material effects and the assumptions concerning social action it inspires. In particular, I want to question the idea of a definite technological watershed in terms of identities and social relations, particularly those that concern new conditions for sexual practice in relation to technologies such as HIV treatment. In this regard, I want to draw on the work of analysts who have depicted the history of the HIV epidemic as dynamic and entwined with bio-technological innovation. I also want to make note of how HIV medical technologies can mediate public health governance, but also how these effects can be engaged with on a dialogical basis.

It is possible to argue that the history of HIV is dynamic and has always involved bio-technological knowledge and effects. Paula Treichler has pointed out how watershed notions of the HIV epidemic were prefigured in its foundational discourse:

> At the same time that "AIDS" is new, however, it is always already occupied, peopled with discourse that predated it and establishing precedent for language not yet invented. The proclamations since 1996 that "AIDS is over" or that "the cure" has been found must likewise be read from this discursive trajectory (Treichler, 1999: 323–324).

Treichler noted how a 1992 book called *AIDS: the making of a chronic disease,* anticipated an unrealised treatment context (Treichler, 1999: see page 325). Research of news media over the course of the 1990s, the period that coincided with the advent of HIV treatment, has revealed changes in the dominant discourses, from 'AIDS as death sentence' to a discourse of hope through bio-technology (Lupton, 1998). Simon Watney has argued for an account of the HIV epidemic that engages with its dynamic qualities. Watney noted that: "Most people no longer speak of AIDS as a crisis. It has become part of the general social and mental furniture of our times" (2000: 260). Eric Rofes used the idea of 'living after crisis' to characterise the HIV prevention concerns of the 1990s compared with those of the 1980s (1999). Rofes referred to the "... emerging cultures" of gay men in the late 1990s and of "... community beyond crisis" (1998: 28). In their research of gay communities living inside and outside the large urban centres most affected by the HIV epidemic, Dowsett and colleagues used the term 'post-AIDS' to denote the shifting social contexts of risk subjectivity in relation to the history of HIV, and not HIV treatment alone (2001). Dowsett and colleagues were concerned to elaborate on new educational agendas for effective HIV prevention:

> By 'post-AIDS' we mean a fragmentation and multiplication of gay community responses to HIV/AIDS, a differentiation in both experiences and consequences that warranted a new, multifaceted approach to health education among gay men, whether HIV-positive or negative (2001: 209).

This idea of post-AIDS needs to be distinguished from the concept of 'living after crisis': "Post-AIDS describes a more detailed configuration of the lives of gay men and shifts in their disposition toward sex, sociality and community" (2001: 209). In these perspectives, including 'post-AIDS', technological change is managed by active subjects interested in finding and using bio-technological, political, social and personal strategies for dealing with the epidemic. Transition is less about 'before and after' and more about dynamic techno-social action made by active subjects.

There is also some ambiguity regarding the material effects of HIV treatment and related technologies on the risk of HIV transmission, that have implications for public health governance. For example, in contrast with fears that HIV treatment may lead to a post-treatment epidemic of HIV, there are several ways in which HIV treatment can be used to prevent HIV transmission. The most notable of these is the use of short-term HIV treatment around birth to inhibit infection of the baby (Alcorn, 2002). Short-term HIV treatment can also be used to prevent HIV infection after sex without condoms (Korner et al., 2006). There is also evidence that treatment can reduce the chance of HIV transmission in sexual practice in treated populations (Porco et al., 2004).

HIV medical technologies also have a property of extending public health governance as a matter of self-discipline. Brian Heaphy has argued that: "... we need to account for experiences where AIDS/HIV can appear both to empower and discipline individuals" (1996: 159). In this view, HIV treatment itself has governmental properties:

> ... it must be acknowledged that while the multiplication of expert systems that mediate different AIDS/HIV knowledges may appear to open up choice, this multiplication may also be indicative of both the expansion of judges of normality and the extension of disciplining discourses (1996: 158).

Heaphy suggested that the proliferation of bio-technology in the area of HIV realises an expanding duality of choices and regulatory requirements. Also in this line of argument, Kane Race has suggested that: "... it is necessary to look at how technological change creates and sustains new selves and bodies, new political technologies and institutes an ongoing process of othering" (2001: 177). Race has addressed one particular aspect of HIV bio-technology, the viral load blood test. The test provides an index of the amount of HIV in the body and is used to infer viral activity (Pozniak et al., 2001). Race considered how HIV viral load testing can be used to determine if the person has been adhering to their treatment prescription. The viral load test is therefore a: "... tool that links matters of individual and public health" (2001: 168). Joined with the HIV antibody test, the viral load test is therefore implicated in the regulation of the sexual relations of the patient in terms of the containment of HIV. Race's perspective suggests that aside from questions concerning whether the risk knowledge provided by bio-technologies has a role in increasing risky practice, the same bio-technologies are implicated in making risky practice observable in new ways and moreover, multiplying the putative risky conduct on the part of people with HIV.

It is also the case that HIV treatment itself is a mediated practice that relies on the relationship between individuals and prescribers. In this sense, HIV treatment resembles other technologically intensive forms of health care, for example, cancer (Delvecchio-Good, 2001). This was the terrain addressed by Flowers, myself and colleagues in a study funded as part of the United Kingdom ESRC Innovative Health technologies Programme called 'Transitions in HIV' (*york.ac.uk/res/iht/* accessed 10 August 2008). One of our interviewees put the experience of treatment this way:

> I'm well aware of the risks that are involved ... ... to keep on top of those risks I have myself monitored more often and make sure I know the results and what have you. And when the time comes we can go back on. But in the meantime we always try and find a solution to whatever's caused the problem and I've had to go off them. I was having breaks from therapy long before it was sort of accepted. It was a definite no-no and other people including friends and other doctors, apart from my main doctor, were very sceptical and didn't think it was a good idea. But as I say I'm very fortunate that Doctor X is brilliant. He really is. We do work as a team and it's never been a problem. He always tells me about stuff I don't know and it's never been a problem
> I: So would you say that you work together to come up with solutions?
> R: Yes, yes.
> I: And you obviously read material and do research outside what...
> R: I'm not obsessed by it, but if there's something new coming up I'll have a read. I may not necessarily remember at all but at least I've had some background. If something's wrong with me that I'm not familiar with I'll go on the net and find out or read something about it ... (Davis et al., 2006a: 337)

Other researchers have made similar arguments. Asha Persson and colleagues have addressed viral load and other blood tests in relation to patient experience (2003). They argue for: "... technologically-mediated negotiation within patient experience" (2003: 397). Although knowledge derived from bio-technologies are not the only forms of knowledge incorporated into self-care, technologies such as viral load test sit at the interface of patient and expert knowledges. Because doctors and patients may not share the same way of thinking about health and illness, the viral load test results and other clinical markers become important technological mediations of self-care and clinical expertise. As Persson and colleagues pointed out:

> ... health is construed and negotiated in relation to medical technology, alternative health models, social embeddedness and bodily experiences. Seen from this perspective, health and illness are always contested rather than coherent, always emergent and changeable rather than determined. Health meanings, therefore never really reach the point of finality, but circulate within an ongoing, shifting dialogue between professional discourses, public narratives and personal lifeworlds, and are mobilised at different points along an illness trajectory to make experiences and actions intelligible to self and others (2003: 411).

For Persson and colleagues, this situated, technological mediation of the patient-prescriber relationship necessarily gives rise to collaborative, dialogical methods for engaging with the knowledge systems that underpin HIV bio-technologies.

The treatment optimism narrative

Despite critical perspectives regarding determinism provided by the notion of a dynamic HIV epidemic entwined with bio-technological innovation, and the regulatory but dialogical properties of such bio-technologies, much research has focused on the impact of treatment on sexual practice. This research focus is most clearly expressed in the concept of 'treatment optimism'. This is the idea that hopeful beliefs and perceptions regarding the effectiveness of HIV treatment might lead people to give up safer sex. As the following discussion will reveal, the treatment optimism idea is not a particularly useful way of explaining the relationship between HIV bio-technologies and sexual practice. Nevertheless, it is worth considering the treatment optimism thesis for several reasons. Despite its limitations, treatment optimism has acquired a taken-for-granted status in HIV prevention research and policy. In relation to cancer, Mary-Jo Delvecchio-Good has noted how clinical narratives of healing provide methods for organising the burgeoning knowledge derived from the science and technology that supports treatment (2001). I want to suggest that treatment optimism provides a narrative that organises and summarises the relationship between HIV bio-technologies and sexual practice that is consistent with public health rationalities of technological determinism. Treatment optimism also works as a way of focussing the problem of governing individuals in the situation of treatment innovation, with specific reference to the rational use of knowledge derived from bio-technologies. It provides a way of addressing the knowledgeable user of HIV bio-technologies and placing them at the centre of public health strategies for the post-treatment situation. This expectation of knowledgeability is reflected in various policy statements. For example, the British HIV Association guidelines recommend that treatment users should "... have knowledge of their results" including viral load and drug-resistant virus tests (Gazzard, 2005: 6). This is also the premise of internet-based treatment information services (see *aidsmap.org* in the United Kingdom and *thebody.com* in the United States, both accessed 10 August 2008).

Research has used forced choice surveys to investigate treatment optimism and sexual practice. This methodology addresses knowledge and beliefs and relies on an assumption that to some extent expectations of effective HIV treatment, such as reduced infectiousness and improved life expectations and therefore reduced fear of either HIV infection or its health consequences, have led to increased risk behaviour. It is derived from measures of agreement with statements such as: "New medical treatments for HIV/AIDS make safer sex less important than it was", "AIDS is now very nearly cured", "Safer sex is as important now as ever" (Kelly et al., 1998: F93); and "People with undetectable viral load do not need to worry so much about infecting others with HIV", "New treatments will take the worry out of sex", "Until there is a complete cure for HIV/AIDS, prevention is still the best practice" (van de Ven et al., 2000: 176).

Elford has summarised the findings of treatment optimism research (2006). There does appear to be empirical support for an association between treatment expectations and risky sexual behaviour among gay men. However, Elford has cautioned that an association is not directional. It may be that gay men who know their sexual practice has possibly exposed them to HIV risk may rely on the idea of treatment optimism as an *ex post facto* anxiety-reduction strategy. Elford argued that treatment optimism research is therefore "unresolved" (Elford, 2006: 27). He also argued that since most gay men are realistic concerning HIV risk in relation to HIV bio-technologies, only a small amount of the increase in risky sex can be attributed to concepts such as treatment optimism. This analysis helps to question the idea that bio-technologies influence sexual practice in a simple manner.

Part of the problem with treatment optimism as an explanation for sexual practice and HIV bio-technologies is related to its conceptual origins in aspects of health psychology and in particular, the Health Belief Model (HBM). The HBM is itself derived from public health attempts to engage with technological innovation. According to Irwin Rosenstock, the model was developed in the 1950s as a way of explaining why some people did not take up screening tests for TB, rheumatic fever, polio and influenza (1974). Apparently, up to that point, public health researchers had thought of themselves as working to prevent disease and had therefore not been involved in treatment. Rosenstock argued that changes in knowledge of diseases, new treatments and diagnostic technologies meant that the margins of prevention and treatment were blurred. In crude terms, the HBM posits that a feared stimulus will be avoided. For HIV prevention, this means that fear of infection motivates safer sex. When fear of HIV infection reduces, such as in light of effective HIV treatment, it follows that motivation to do safer sex will also subside.

This HBM-related model for safer sex has been widely criticised. The HBM model arose in an era when public health was not questioned and in the context of policies of universal right to health care provision and the related functionalist assumptions of benign medical paternalism and required patient altruism. Researchers have argued that a resort to fear motivation models of health behaviour in relation to sexual health and HIV are likely to be ineffective because they promote an understanding of HIV infection as shameful and a source of stigma (Slavin et al., 2007). In addition, the idea that fear motivates risk avoidance is not particularly relevant for people who know they have HIV infection, or suspect they may have it, a problem that has not typically been a focus in survey research and which may supply a crucial explanation for the limitations of the findings regarding treatment optimism. A central problem with the HBM concerns how it assumes that social actors are calculating and risk-averse individuals. Such individualism associates risky behaviour with conceptions of volition and psychological processes, so that the person becomes a focus for intervention, as opposed to social or institutional practices. In this regard, there is a striking resemblance with the preoccupations in much e-dating research, which also conflates practice with individual behaviour. However, this arrangement is useful for public health governance because it assumes that the link between technology and risky sex is mediated by individuals themselves. In this sense, individuals become the conduits of risk and the focus for intervention.

Perhaps the most well known critique of risk individualism is that developed by Mary Douglas (1992). Douglas argued that individualising approaches to risk are forensic in the sense that, despite being overtly scientised, they nevertheless provide the means for apportioning blame. In Douglas's cultural theory of risk, the forensic identities of social agents become important: "To be 'at risk' is equivalent to being sinned against, being vulnerable to the events caused by others, whereas being 'in sin' means being the cause of harm" (1992: 28). This articulation of blame and identity has been discussed in HIV social research. As I have suggested elsewhere, the meanings attached to HIV serostatus bring about unequal responsibilities in risk management, where the person with HIV was seen to have extra responsibilities (Davis, 2002). Other researchers have suggested that people with HIV, through a "... cruel twisting of logic" can be held to blame for the risk of HIV transmission even when the partner decided to have sex without condoms (Cusick & Rhodes, 2000: 481). Quantitative research has suggested that a majority of gay men who are not infected expect their HIV positive partners to disclose their HIV status prior to sex (Reid et al., 2002). Qualitative research has shown that these questions of responsibility translate into deciding whether or not, or how, to disclose HIV status with a sexual partner (Keogh et al., 1995). This practice was shown to be problematic, either if disclosure was achieved, or if it was not. People faced rejection and an intensification of responsibility for the safety of sexual interaction if they disclosed. If people did not disclose, they faced negative feelings such as guilt. Keogh and colleague's research also suggests that the settings of sexual relations are important (1995). For example, casual anonymous sex was seen as a situation that did not require disclosure and where sexual risk was an individual responsibility. However, in the situation where a casual sexual contact turned into a more regular and emotionally important partnership, people faced a dilemma of when to tell if they had not done so at the outset. In research of the impact of treatment on sexual practice, interviewees suggested that the avoidance of the negative social consequences of blame influenced sexual practice:

> I don't want to have it on my conscience that I infected somebody. Because, I wouldn't be able to deal with that very well ... ... That would fuck up more so than any other thing, knowing that I had

actually infected someone, knowing what I do. Now if I did it unintentionally, if the condom broke or something, and it was their choice, they knew I was positive, then there's nothing I can do about that. But if I fucked somebody and knew that I should have used a condom, and they were negative and found out six months down the line that they were positive, I wouldn't be able to deal with that very well (Davis, 2008: in press).

In such accounts, treatment optimism is not relevant. Social actors are concerned with the mitigation of some of the other aspects of HIV prevention concerning blame.

Reflexive HIV treatment

The treatment optimism narrative therefore reveals problems in dominant understandings of bio-technologies and sexual practice. But there is reason to argue for a different narrative of bio-technology, sex and epidemic. This alternative makes different assumptions concerning sexual agency, foregrounding reflexive engagements with the technological mediation of sexual practice. This approach bears some resemblance to the treatment optimism approach because it does concern itself with a knowledgeable actor, engaging with information generated by the blood tests important for HIV treatment. But this approach departs from treatment optimism because it conceptualises sexual agents as capable of, and interested in, making sexual cultures through their own actions, including through the application of bio-technological knowledge and effects.

This notional reflexive HIV treatment has its origins in the politics of treatment access. Prior to the advent of treatable HIV, access to drugs that may have provided some form of moderation of HIV infection was a central question. Treatment advocacy projects were therefore a pronounced aspect of community-based responses to HIV. These projects focused on overcoming bureaucratic and scientific barriers to any possible treatment that might have had some beneficial effects. The advocacy movement also involved the promotion of the involvement of people affected by the epidemic in how treatment science was managed. As such, the advocacy movement revealed a concern with governing access to treatment and how it was to be used. A central premise was what Treichler has called: "… a radical and democratic technoculture" (1999: 280). This premise refers to forms of active engagement with medicine on the part of people affected by HIV, to further access to, and enhance influence over the use of, treatment. As Treichler put it:

> ... the strongest challenge to current conditions comes not from those who dismiss or denounce technology but rather from those who seek a more progressive, intelligent, and participatory deployment of science and scientific theory in everyday life ... ... The strength of their guiding theoretical frame lies not in a resistance to orthodox science but in strategic conceptions of "scientific truth" that leave room for action in the face of contradictions. This makes it possible to seek local, partial solutions and to give more attention to difference and diversity (1999: 298).

This perspective gives rise to a vision of bio-technology as made and applied by people affected by HIV, and those who care for them, in the interests of survival. Treichler also implied that intervention in HIV treatment requires an elaboration of forms of participation in knowledge-making concerning bio-technology, but without relinquishing the capacity to contest truth-making criteria and practices. Steven Epstein has shown how scientific knowledge production in relation to HIV has been subject to the interests of affected communities (1996). Examples include the invention of safer sex and the participation of people with HIV in the management and dissemination of information regarding the clinical trials of treatments. Democratisation of HIV bio-technology then is seen as a basis for articulating forms of social relations that construct and redistribute knowledge in desirable ways, and by implication, including those that pertain to sexual practice.

But Epstein also raised a cautionary note. While activism has helped to reconfigure some aspects of HIV medicine, several forms of re-medicalisation may also occur, in terms of the medical objectification of identity and the reconfiguration of activism (2000). Epstein noted how in an effort to influence the use of HIV bio-technologies, activists themselves have been drawn into medical systems of authority, creating a kind of "expertification" and "... hierarchies of expertise" that may be shaped around, and therefore help to reproduce, health inequalities related to class, gender and ethnicity (Epstein, 2000: web document). He also suggested that the activist inspired focus on the health needs of marginal populations, mostly figured around these categories of class, gender and ethnicity, has a possible unintended by-product of the objectification of such groups in biological terms, creating the prospect that social inequality comes to be understood as a matter of biology. This aspect of medicalisation leads into a kind of reification of bio-technological identity categories, a process that folds back onto HIV activism to create problems for the general project of influencing HIV treatment in desirable ways (Epstein, 2000). This re-medicalisation is a challenge for the idea of techno-democracy, as it suggests that activism, in the effort of reshaping the practice of treatment, returns us to forms of exclusion, strengthened with forms of bio-technological determinism. The re-medicalisation of social categories also seems to be a problem if a democratic form of reflexive treatment is enacted without an epistemological edge. For example, Treichler noted that treatment advocacy needs to acknowledge the provisionalities of the knowledge-making practices of science. But Epstein's account revealed an idealised thread in techno-democracy. In his account there is an unresolved matter of the tensions between democratisation of HIV treatment and bio-technological 'colonisation' of the social.

With reference to sexual practice, researchers have taken the position that the self-aware use of HIV bio-technology, a kind of techno-democracy, has made forms of HIV prevention possible. In the early 1990s, survey findings were interpreted to reveal that gay men used HIV testing and serostatus to make decisions regarding the need for the use of condoms in regular partnerships (Kippax, 1993). HIV negative men in particular were observed to give up condoms with their HIV negative partners. These practices were termed "... negotiated safety" and reflected a reworking of contemporary HIV prevention guidelines of 'use a condom every time' (Kippax, 1993: 257). These practices were seen to exhibit rational application of knowledge connected with the HIV antibody blood test. The idea of negotiated safety was an important break in conceptualising HIV prevention, precisely because it foregrounded agency on the part of gay men in HIV prevention practice. Attending to the post-treatment situation, Sue Kippax has asserted that: "... safer sex culture remains intact BECAUSE, not in spite of the incorporation of medicine into prevention" (authors emphasis 1999: 13). Through negotiated safety, bio-technologies were present in the lives of gay men prior to the advent of effective treatment. Kippax and Race have jointly and independently explored the terms of a "conversation" between gay men's sexual culture and public health, arguing that gay men have continued to elaborate on the relevance of bio-technologies for managing risk in their sexual relationships (Kippax & Race, 2003; Race, 2003: 369).

It also seems possible to argue that HIV bio-technologies mediate social and sexual relations. Paul Flowers has suggested a kind of periodisation of HIV prevention and bio-technology (2001). He has suggested three 'eras': mobilisation; somaticisation; technologisation. The first comprised the early stages of the epidemic characterised by community mobilisation around the notion of safer sex in the context of a lack of scientific understanding of HIV. With the discovery of the HIV pathogen in the early 1980s and therefore the invention of the HIV antibody blood test, a second period emerged to do with 'somaticisation' and 'individualisation'. In this period, risk management was informed by the idea that some people had HIV and some did not, making it possible to distinguish different bodies in relation to HIV prevention. This focus accentuated the importance of the individual management of HIV risk reduction connected with self-knowledge of HIV status. Patti Lather has also addressed the social aspects of the HIV antibody blood test, but in terms of relationality (1995). In Lather's terms, the antibody blood test is a method for defining risk between individuals. It assigns a valency of HIV positive or negative to test results and therefore provides individuals with a relational risk identity, for example + to –, – to –, + to +, – to untested and so on. Lather made the point that HIV transmission risk does not reside in positive or negative identity, but in the difference between them. In this sense, bio-technology is implicated in the construction of risk relationships figured around knowledge of HIV serostatus. Qualitative research in the United Kingdom has suggested that sex between men with HIV or with men who did not have HIV require different risk assessments and negotiations (Keogh et al., 1999). Focus groups with gay men with HIV in 1995, that is, prior to the HIV treatment watershed, revealed that interviewees made connections between HIV diagnostic tests and the risk of HIV transmission: "... when my T cells are below 400, then I know that I'm probably very infectious" (Keogh et al., 1995: 32).

However, Flowers has suggested that the advent of effective HIV treatment and the related technologies used to monitor its effectiveness in individual bodies has disrupted modes of knowledge and prevention figured around HIV antibody serostatus:

> ... now this commonality between bodies and HIV status has been eroded by the advent of new testing technologies which address viral activity (viral load, viral resistance) as changing both temporally and spatially, across disease progression and bodily parts (plasma and semen) (2001: 67).

According to Flowers, these new bio-technologies lead to a "fracturing" of risk management practices, into increasingly technically differentiated and privatised considerations (2001: 63). Researchers in Australia have used qualitative methodologies to explore how HIV bio-technologies might have been associated with risk behaviour among gay men (Rosengarten et al., 2001). These researchers argued that sex with and without condoms was not attributed to "… clinical markers" such as measures of viral load (2001: 10). This perspective underlines the explanatory limitations of the notion of treatment optimism. However, these researchers also argued that gay men with HIV employed "… individually tailored risk minimisation strategies" and that "… undetectable or low viral load may provide for a reduced sense of infectivity" (2001: 4). According to these researchers, gay men with HIV applied knowledge of infectiousness and viral load test results to sexual practice. They deployed epidemiological perspectives such as the relative HIV transmission risk of insertive and receptive sexual intercourse, a practice that has come to be called 'strategic positioning'. Strategic positioning means adopting a position in sexual intercourse that is thought to reduce the risk of HIV transmission. Both disclosure of HIV serostatus or assumptions about it were used to determine the serostatus of the sexual partner, identified as part of a "… pos/pos sub culture" of anal sex without condoms (Rosengarten et al., 2001: 33). This practice has been somewhat reified in the term 'serosorting', now widely used by researchers. Serosorting pertains to having sex without condoms with someone of (or assumed to be) the same HIV antibody status. For example, gay men who know they have HIV might assume the receptive position in sex, which is thought to somewhat reduce HIV transmission. Strategic positioning and serosorting may not be new, and specifically post-HIV treatment, practices. The observation of negotiated safety among gay men in the early 1990s suggests that some gay men have used such bio-technologically informed strategies since the beginning of the epidemic (Kippax, 1993). Rosengarten and colleagues argued that HIV treatment was not leading to the abandonment of safer sex among gay men. However, the social and sexual relations of risk management did seem to be informed by understandings derived from HIV bio-technology, including its changing effects.

It also appears that engagements with HIV bio-technologies are diverse and complex and in part reliant on the ongoing 'conversation' between bio-technology users and experts (Kippax & Race, 2003). In research conducted by colleagues and myself in the United Kingdom, interviewees depicted HIV bio-technologies as necessarily concerning questions of expertise (Davis et al., 2002). Such resort to expertise was an important strategy for dealing with the contentious and debatable implications of HIV bio-technologies for HIV transmission, such as the concept of reinfection with drug-resistant forms of HIV. In the following account, the interviewee refers to negotiation between himself and his sexual partner regarding the need for condoms in their sexual relationship:

> ... we both spoke to our doctors ... we'd made a decision within the months that we're going to have a monogamous relationship, and there was a lot of talk then about ... the possibilities of cross-infection ... the issues of drug resistance weren't applicable because neither of us had ever taken any of the drugs ... neither of our doctors, who are both very well versed and experienced in HIV medicine ... said that it wouldn't be a problem. They said there may be some risks but it seems unlikely because it's not like [we] have different strains ... so their feeling was that as long as we were both absolutely sure that we were being faithful to each other then it ... wasn't going to cause a problem ... so it was up to us. And so we chose that we wouldn't use condoms ... (Davis et al., 2002: 38).

In this account, medical authority makes an appearance in the negotiation of the use of condoms in sexual practice. Medical experts are represented as superlative sources of knowledge and advice regarding the implications of HIV-biotechnologies for the risk of HIV transmission. Such a narrative strategy indicates that engagements with medical expertise underpin the implications of bio-technology for sexual practice. In the next account, the interviewee depicts a more independent engagement with the knowledge systems of HIV bio-technologies:

> ... I think it's slightly irresponsible to run the risk of reinfection ... My own reading of the literature on this is that nobody has established that reinfection occurs but they believe that there is a significant risk of reinfection with the two doses of HIV, one of which may be resistant to your current drug regime ... I don't want to myself in a situation where ... I get a viral load back and my CD4 count starts to drop, because I think those things will be quite hard to handle emotionally ... (Davis et al., 2002: 39).

Both these accounts provide a contrast with the treatment optimism narrative. They reveal reflexivity with regard to HIV bio-technology, related uncertainties, and implications for sexual practice. They suggest new questions regarding how we understand the relationship between bio-technologies and sexual practice, such as the social relations of expertise and the complexities of HIV treatment itself. But it seems that complexity itself may also be challenging:

> ... I just believe HIV is HIV ... I know there are different strains out there and I don't wish to contemplate too much, because a lot of it's to do with luck and I've been one of the lucky ones ... If you get a really bad strain where it knocks you off your perch in two years, well it's just luck ... There's not much more that can go wrong once you've already got ... it (Davis et al., 2002: 37).

In this account, an engagement with bio-technological complexity is swept aside. The strategy is purified of uncertainty and turns to a foundational strategy for addressing the implications of HIV treatment that is derived from the HIV antibody blood test and its categorical notions of HIV positive and HIV negative. It represents a turning back to a pre-treatment ordering of HIV risk subjectivity, a strategy that is not properly acknowledged by the concept of treatment optimism and other deterministic notions of the relationships between HIV bio-technologies and sexual practice.

Hyper-technologisation and sexual cultures

HIV bio-technologies, HIV prevention and sexual culture form a dense network of connections and interdependencies. This complexity is revealed in the research I have discussed concerning the reflections of gay men on their sexual practice in light of the effects of HIV bio-technologies. Central practices in this regard appear to be strategic positioning and serosorting which both reflect the application of HIV bio-technological knowledge to sexual practice. In addition, it is possible to argue that internet-mediated partnering has a significant role to play in such complexity. As I have discussed in the previous chapter, e-dating websites rely on technology that lends itself to the coding of aspects of self, such as appearance and sexual interests. Such coding of the self extends to knowledge made available by other forms of technology that derive categories, in particular HIV serostatus. In this section, I want to consider internet-mediated serosorting and how it is mobilised by requirements concerning HIV prevention. I want to use this example to flesh out the concept of hyper-technologisation. In Chapter 1, I referred to the example of the *Safe Sex Passport* which allowed e-daters to display their sexual health status for prospective partners, in a way that expresses a general public health rationality of clean/unclean or cordon sanitaire (Waldby et al., 1993). Some gay men's e-dating sites are constructed so that users can indicate whether or not they practice safer sex (*gaydar.com* accessed 10 August 2008) and their HIV serostatus (*manhunt.net* accessed 10 August 2008). These uses of websites reflect the coding property built into internet technology. They also inspire a vision of social relating mediated by bio- and communication technology, and in the present context, a form of public health governance, that is systematically predetermined, or hyper-technologised. This notional systematisation of sexual relations may explain some of its attraction both for its practitioners and public health governance. Such practices help insert public health rationalities into sexual cultures. They reflect a specific intensification of the emergence of patterns of sexual and social interaction according to bio-technological characteristics, giving rise to a kind of cybernetic public health. But I will argue that this new form of public health governance may be mythical. HIV serostatus made literal on websites and as the basis for serosorting as prevention relies on a constant and universal regime of testing for HIV and sexually transmitted infections. The cost of such testing alone would inhibit such approaches to disease control. But the approach also trades on a utopian vision of a thoroughly hybridised public health, technology and sexual relating. It therefore extends a mythical public health governance derived from deterministic understandings of technosexuality.

Epidemiological research has investigated engagements with HIV bio-technologies expressed as strategic positioning and serosorting. Evidence for serosorting has been found in surveys of gay men in New York (Halkitis et al., 2007), San Francisco (Osmond et al., 2007), London (Elford et al., 2007), Amsterdam (Van der Bij et al., 2007), and Sydney (Mao et al., 2006). Researchers have reported that internet-based male sex workers in the United States have adopted strategic positioning with their commercial sex partners (Bimbi & Parsons, 2007). Research among Latino gay men with HIV in Boston, New York and Washington has found that same serostatus partnerships were the most likely to have anal sex without condoms (Poppen et al., 2005). Longitudinal research over the period of 1998–2005 in London found evidence for serosorting (Elford et al., 2007). Looking at the serosorting paradigm another way, researchers in Seattle found that people with HIV, that is both gay men and heterosexual people, reported that sexual partners had chosen to not have sex with them because of their HIV serostatus (Golden et al., 2007). Research with gay men who do not use condoms, that is, the so-called barebackers, found that these men employed both strategic positioning and serosorting to reduce the risk of HIV transmission (Grov et al., 2007). Survey data from gay men in Australia over the period of 1996 to 2003, shows a gradual relaxation of condom use and an increase in strategic positioning (Van De Ven et al., 2004). These changes are taken as evidence of bio-technologically informed harm reduction among gay men, although these researchers are careful to acknowledge that strategic positioning is not as effective as condom use.

Elford has made the point that these harm reduction strategies are associated, and in a sense made more systematic, with the use of the internet (2006). As I noted in the previous chapter, qualitative research in London has shown that gay men with HIV can use forms of internet-based communication, such as their online profiles, chat or messaging to indicate their HIV serostatus (Davis et al., 2006c). Researchers in the United States have also considered how so-called barebackers use the internet to find suitable partners (Carballo-Dieguez et al., 2006). Other researchers in the United States conducted a content analysis of the online profiles of gay men who identified as 'gift givers' and 'bug chasers', that is, seeking to spread HIV and be infected by HIV, respectively (Grov & Parsons, 2006). These researchers found that only a small proportion revealed that they intended to have sex that would transmit HIV. A substantial minority were actually seeking men of the same serostatus, in apparent contradiction of their supposed self labels of bug chaser or gift giver. However, most were seen to be ambivalent in relation to the serostatus of their prospective partner, perhaps a reflection of assumptions concerning the online contexts provided by the barebacking websites. Other researchers have made similar observations. For instance, it has been suggested that one of the reasons gay men with HIV attended barebacking sex parties was "... relief from burdens of serostatus disclosure" (Clatts et al., 2005: 373). Race has argued that barebacking may be a form of code for HIV positive serostatus and therefore a form of serosorting, explaining the apparent ambivalence of gay men who use bareback websites to find sexual partners (2003). Using barebacking websites may therefore be a form of safer sex that flows from the logic of serosorting and through it, the logic of the risk relationship produced by HIV antibody serostatus, as mentioned earlier. Ironically, the apparently outrageous use of barebacking websites is itself derived from the combination of HIV bio-technologies and the imperative of HIV prevention.

However, Race also admitted that such HIV prevention strategies are fragile and open to errors that have to do with, what he referred to as, disparities in knowledge and 'sexual capital'. Picking up Race's point regarding fragility, the flaws in barebacking as HIV prevention have been addressed by Barry Adam (2005). In research concerning bare-backing and internet communication, Adam has argued that barebackers rely on an ethical stance of HIV prevention that draws on the atomising of the social agency embedded in neo-liberalism. In particular, Adam has said that barebacking is supported by the notion of caveat emptor, which implies that each sexual actor is expected to be knowledgeable in their actions and personally responsible for harm to themselves. Adam argues that such practices may lead to mistaken assumptions among those who do not subscribe to such ethical frameworks or simply fail to comprehend them. The caveat emptor approach appears to contradict the relational ethics discussed by cyber-feminists and found at the heart of debates concerning sexual citizenship and HIV prevention. Several commentators have questioned whether the practice of barebacking/serosorting is at all tenable as a method of HIV prevention. Researchers argue that because people may not know they are infected and believe themselves to be HIV negative, serosorting may actually work to increase HIV transmission (Butler & Smith, 2007).

There are also problems in the ways in which practices such as sero-sorting are framed in public health discourse. Researchers are assuming that people serosort to pursue the public health imperative of HIV prevention. But preventing HIV may not be the only justification for such practices. Research from France compared the reasons for risky sex among HIV positive heterosexual and homosexual people (Peretti-Watel et al., 2006). These researchers made the argument that risky sex reflects how sexual practice is culturally organised. For women with HIV, most of whom arrived in France from Africa, sexual practice was influenced by their relative lack of power in their steady heterosexual partnership. For heterosexual men, risky sex was associated with dislike of condoms with a steady partner. For gay men, risky sex was associated with 'casual sex'. While research such as this relies on crude notions of sexual practice and its associated social aspects, it does remind us that the cultural organisation of sexual practice provides the main context for behaviours that might transmit HIV and sexually transmitted infections. As I have indicated in previous sections, people may not serosort in order to fulfil expectations regarding HIV prevention in the narrow sense. The blaming attached to HIV positive serostatus may be an important, or even the most important, aspect of the practice. It may also be that serosorting means different things depending on self-knowledge of HIV sero-status. It is important to recognise these provisions on the notion of serosorting as a method of HIV prevention. For example, in some public health writing, serosorting is coming to be understood as a form of quarantine that resonates with the notion of cordon sanitaire in HIV prevention. For example, researchers have begun to distinguish between the "... self-protecting attitudes of HIV-negative men" and the "... partner-protecting attitudes of HV-positive men" (Patel et al., 2006: 1046). Serosorting is therefore seen as self-protective among HIV negative men but as an altruistic duty among gay men with HIV. The prospect that gay men with HIV might serosort to protect themselves from blame is not properly considered in such approaches.

Conclusion

In this chapter, I have developed an account of hyper-technologisation with reference to bio- and communication technologies. This chapter has therefore built on the previous one concerning e-dating and sexual health. I have expanded the concept of technosexuality to incorporate bio-technologies and their hybridisation with the internet, with particular reference to practices such as, so-called, internet-mediated serosorting. I have pointed out how research concerning both e-dating and HIV bio-technologies has subscribed to assumptions of determinism. Such approaches are rather limited because they ignore the cultural aspects of sexual practice. These approaches also make an assumption concerning agency that relies on notions of individualised, rational action and risk aversion. In this regard, the HBM, and its expression in the concept of treatment optimism, was used as an example. I also considered how the concept of treatment optimism, despite its explanatory limitations, endures because it provides a powerful organising strategy for governing the intersection of HIV bio-technologies and sexual cultures. It may also endure because its individualising qualities have a forensic property that permits the assignment of blame for HIV transmission.

In place of treatment optimism, I have argued for an alternative that recognises the self-conscious action on the part of sexual agents. This point of view avoids some of the problems of determinism because it attends to the ways in which people make HIV bio-technologies work in terms of their sexual practices. Key examples of this view are the democratic underpinnings of HIV treatment advocacy, the social relations of expertise that are necessarily part of the considerations of HIV bio-technologies in sexual practice, and internet-mediated serosorting. In addition, I have argued that internet-mediated serosorting is achieved through the ways in which the internet furnishes methods for coding the sexual body, intentions and bio-technological knowledge such as

HIV serostatus. Extending the argument I made in the previous chapter, internet-mediated serosorting gives visibility to the ways in which bio-technologies are being taken into sexual practice. It also points to the ways in which public health is itself involved in hyper-technologisation, suggesting the emergence of mediatised and bio-technologised public health sociality. Although many of my examples are derived from research with gay and other homosexually-interested men, this theory of hyper-technologisation is likely to be a useful perspective for reflecting on public the health governance of sexually transmitted infections and HIV in general.

These last two chapters have therefore worked to argue for a view of technosexuality that keeps society and technology in play. A key theme in this regard has been the ways in which forms of public health rationality influence how the sexual health implications of e-dating and HIV bio-technologies are understood and also how they can be combined. This perspective also supplies a way of interrogating the limitations of public health assumptions regarding sexual agency, such as assuming that people with HIV serosort only because it affords some form of reduction of the risk of HIV transmission. A related concept here concerns the underlying assumption of risk aversion that gives rise to a HIV negative-centrism expressed in the notions that HIV negative gay men serosort as an act of self-protection, while HIV positive gay men serosort to protect others. Such notions seem quite functionalist and over-determined in light of the relational ethics regarded as central to the life politics of technosexual citizenship. These critiques extend Halperin's argument I used in Chapter 1, concerning the psycho-pathologisation of gay men in public health research. But in the present case, it is the involvement of public health in the formation of hyper-technologisation that warrants further scrutiny.

In the next three chapters, I want to deepen this interrogation of technosexuality and public health governance by developing themes identified in these case studies. Building on the critique of techno-determinism and the assumptions it mobilises regarding sexual agency and technology, I want to further reflect on how social action is conceptualised in forms of public health governance. Based on the reversal of the anonymity thesis into what I have called strategic visibility, I want to consider the case for an argument that technosexual visibility supplies an epistemic strategy for public health governance. In relation to the ways in which public health governance is trying to exploit techno-sexuality as the means of extending itself, I want to consider questions of medicalisation.

Therefore, the next chapter turns to public health itself and provides a more detailed exploration of the origins and expression of key imperatives on sexual agency such as altruism, contagion, and risk, and forensics. This chapter will show how public health governance is itself open to contestation over how best to govern epidemics of sexually transmitted infections and HIV. It will also argue that such contestation inhibits a proper engagement with questions of technosexual citizenship, such as relational ethics. The following chapter addresses the theme of visibility and develops it in connection with both bio- and communication technologies. A key aspect of this chapter will be the moral panics regarding forms of internet-mediated sexual practice, such as barebacking. The last substantive chapter in this book explores wider questions of the medicalisation of intimate life and sexual health. A key argument in this regard will be the ways in which technosexuality articulated with public health governance is implicated in the decentring of medical authority in the exercise of sexual health care.

5
Innovation and Imperative

It is plain that public health has an interest in forms of technosexuality, either as a source of danger or as a method for extending itself. In this chapter, I want to address some of the tensions for public health governance concerning the assumptions it relies on regarding the individual and their social relations. In particular I want to address altruism, contagion, risk and forensics. Each of these concepts represents an assumption of social action that finds expression in public health. I also want to consider how technological innovations, particularly of the biological kind, have influenced the expression of these assumptions. In the previous chapter in connection with the Health Belief Model (HBM) and treatment optimism research concerning HIV biotechnologies, I noted some of the effects of assumptions that social actors in the technosexual realm are risk averse and rational individuals. I noted how this assumption of risk aversion may not relate very well with the perspectives of people who already know they have HIV infection. Such assumptions also appear to have a forensic quality because they mobilise blame. In relation to the practice of serosorting, I also made reference to a reliance on altruism and self-protection and how these articulated with the knowledge of HIV embodiment provided by the HIV antibody test. In this chapter, I want to consider if this heterogeneity of risk aversion, altruism and self-protection gives rise to an effective melange of governmental strategies or a muddle of incoherent, and sometimes clashing, assumptions.

It is the case that problems of public health governance in general have been the subject of debate and reflection. For example, a review conducted by the Nuffield Council on Bioethics in the United Kingdom addressed public health governance in relation to infectious diseases, among other concerns (2007). The review sought to reflect on contemporary public health challenges such as SARS, along with older health concerns such as sexually transmitted infections and HIV. The review aimed to clarify how governments should act in relation to such challenges for the good of public health. Drawing on liberal political philosophy, the authors advocated a stewardship model for the government of public health, as opposed to other approaches, such as a custodial one. In this stewardship model, public health institutions should strike a balance between the minimisation of harm and constraints on the rights of the individual to privacy, self-determination, consent, and freedom from coercion. They argued however that the public good does outweigh the rights of the individual or communities, therefore creating a mandate for institutional action with regard to health concerns. But they also acknowledged that action should always be conducted with reference to the particularities of the health concerns and the social circumstances of those affected. In this regard, the stewardship model seems to provide scope for entertaining a social justice approach to sexual health. However, this stewardship model leaves much room for debate and negotiation with regard to how public health should proceed. It also suggests that public health action will necessarily be heterogeneous, or at least, accord with the circumstances of the health concern in question.

In contrast with this stewardship model, it appears that intrusive and universalising forms of public health policy are being considered for technosexuality. Public health practitioners have argued for compliance interventions in e-dating websites, based on the methods of tobacco control (Levine & Klausner, 2005). As I noted in Chapter 1, there are examples of sexual health websites for young people produced in different languages. E-dating websites for gay men already carry banners and pop-ups encouraging e-daters to test for sexually transmitted infections. Importantly however, for the most part these strategies rely on voluntarism, particularly in relation to people running the commercial websites and their subscribers. However, the compliance based approach would see the regulation of commercial e-dating websites for the pursuit of sexual health, including: taxing them and using the funds to develop interventions; and requiring that the websites carry health hazard warnings, health education advertising, and sexual health advice. Complying websites would be given a sexual health 'seal of approval'. Strikingly, the authors also advocated that websites should include sexual health descriptor fields in online profiles so that e-daters can indicate their health status, including information regarding their history of sexually transmitted infections, HIV serostatus, genital herpes and warts (Levine & Klausner, 2005: 55). I have noted how such approaches suggest the notion of cordon sanitaire that Waldby and colleagues used to characterise the clean/unclean sexual partner choice strategies of young heterosexual men (1993). The 'seal of approval' for e-dating websites and online sexual health descriptor fields resonate rather strongly with cordon sanitaire. Strategies such as these also demonstrate how the internet can be used to make public health subjects visible. By formalising and extending the practices of internet-mediated serosorting, they incorporate them into a more general approach to disease control. As I have already noted, such approaches reveal the affinity of forms of public health rationality and the features of internet technologies that are employed in e-dating websites. It is also possible to argue that the concern surrounding technosexuality serves to make it necessary to intervene in such ways, and gives extra impetus for the compliance approach. Public health needs to retain the idea that the internet, Viagra or HIV bio-technologies are dangerous in order to justify the exercise of its authority.

As I have suggested in previous chapters, the compliance approach has problems. Such an approach assumes universal testing for sexually transmitted infections and HIV. It also indicates how public health rationalities are themselves implicated in the shaping of sexual relations. It assumes that sexual interaction is only derived from e-dating websites, when we know from the various cyber-ethnographies that sexual meetings can be facilitated in places such as online game environments, social networking sites and even academic e-lists. So far, the compliance approach has not clearly defined how complying e-dating websites should be regulated and if subscribers will also be required to comply with such regulation. A major problem is also likely to be the stigma of having a sexually transmitted infection or HIV. For example, researchers have shown that people with sexually transmitted infections are perceived as lacking moral judgement (Young et al., 2007). These researchers argued that people avoid the stigma of sexually transmitted infections because they expect social devaluation. Such stigma is likely to discourage people from displaying their test results if they have an infection.

The examples of the stewardship and compliance approaches suggest that public health governance is not necessarily internally consistent or at least that approaches to technosexuality are in the process of being negotiated. In the following therefore, I want to consider theories of self and society that underpin public health governance, that is, altruism, contagion, risk and forensics. While some of these perspectives are outmoded in their pure form, I will show how traces of their legacy remain in forms of public health addressing aspects of technosexuality. I will also discuss technological innovation in relation to these assumptions. I will create an argument that public health governance applied to technosexuality is mixed and open to the deepening of health subjectivity understood in bio-technological terms.

Gift and contagion

To understand public health imperatives we need to consider their origins. The gift relationship is often used as the basis for understanding how public health works. It is a concept that comes out of functionalist sociology. It assumes that reciprocal giving, and through it, the obligations of the individual to society, is necessary for the functioning of society. Another example of functionalism is Talcott Parsons's notion of the sick role. The HBM I discussed in Chapter 4 in connection with HIV bio-technologies, can be taken to have origins in a functionalist view of public health. Also relying on functionalist ideas, Richard Titmuss famously used the example of blood donation as reciprocal giving to develop a theory of altruistic social care. Such models of social organisation have been displaced by theories of reflexivity and governmentality. But it is possible to argue that traces of functionalism expressed in terms of the gift relationship and therefore the obligations of the individual to society inform the operation of public health. It is also the case that the reciprocal giving implied in public health is deeply compromised in several ways. The questions of contagion implied by sexually transmitted infections give special emphasis to obligations to others. The logic of disease control that pervades public health interventions gives rise to identities that reflect the logic of the control of contagion but that sit awkwardly with sexual cultures. In addition, new bio-technologies are also changing the meaning of 'giving to strangers' in ways that appear to be accentuating forms of social exclusion on the grounds of biological characteristics. This tension between an underlying functionalist gift orientation in public health and its reformulation and disruption goes some way to explain the challenges faced in the area of technosexuality and public health governance.

Marcel Mauss's famous 1920s account of the gift relationship is often taken as a starting point for discussion of reciprocal giving (1990 [1950]). Mauss provided many examples of the gift relationship in his summary of ethnographic research with American Indian, Inuit, Polynesian and Melanesian societies. These societies used the giving of made objects, food, festivals and even people, to reinforce and create ties of mutual obligation. In these social systems, the gift is more than just a material object. The gift is seen to retain something of the soul or essence of the giver and create an obligation that the receiver should reciprocate by returning a gift carefully judged to reinforce social ties. The gift has to be reciprocated because to not do so gives too much power to the giver. But equally, giving back too much or too little can shame or belittle givers and receivers and therefore damage social relations. According to Mauss, these systems of reciprocal giving spread in ripples of mutual obligation that help societies to function in a relatively harmonious way. Mauss also suggested that modern societies (for him at least) incorporate gift economies. Indeed, Slater, discussed in Chapter 2, regarded reciprocal giving as the foundation of the social organisation of sex pic trading (2002). However, Mauss also recognised a tension between autonomy and the gift relationship in modern societies. Reflecting on his own European society, Mauss observed:

> Society is seeking to rediscover a cellular structure for itself. It is indeed wanting to look after the individual. Yet the mental state in which it does so is one in which are curiously intermingled a perception of the rights of the individual and other, purer sentiments: charity, social service, and solidarity. The themes of the gift, of the freedom and the obligation inherent in the gift, of generosity and self interest that are linked in giving, are reappearing ... (1990 [1950]: 68).

Mauss therefore presaged a tension created by the rise of individualism and the social good, but in a way that expressed hope for reconciliation.

Drawing on this Maussian notion of reciprocal giving, Titmuss conducted a study of blood donation in the late 1960s (1970). Titmuss compared blood donation policies that relied on payment of the donor, such as in the United States, with voluntary donation, such as in the United Kingdom. Titmuss showed how blood donation was a mix of altruism and self-interest. Giving blood is good for others because it helps them in medical emergencies. It is also good for the self, because giving implies the same treatment at some time in the future (or so the theory goes). However, blood donation differs from Mauss's notion of gift because it is impersonal and there are no immediate requirements of reciprocation.

Titmuss also raised the issue of the contamination of the blood supply by viruses such as hepatitis. When Titmuss was writing his book, there was no blood test for hepatitis (Titmuss, 1970: 25). The only way of preventing hepatitis coming into the blood supply was by asking potential donors questions regarding their medical history and behaviour. Titmuss argued that the safety of the blood supply therefore relied on the potential donor telling the truth. In situations where donations receive payment, donors were seen to be more likely to omit details of their history to avoid being excluded and missing out on financial reward. Conversely, where donation is voluntary, so the theory goes, donors have no incentive to hide the truth. Titmuss argued that voluntary donation helped to prevent the contamination of the blood supply, and by extension, was the ideal approach for social relations in general. Such assumptions concerning the individual and their social relations can be seen in modern public health. For example, the focus on anonymity with regard to internet-mediated sexual practices, particularly in relation to self-knowledge of sexually transmitted infections, resembles Titmuss's concerns with truth and the contamination of the blood supply.

Mauss's theory of gift is reciprocal, embodied and face-to-face. Blood donation is impersonal and mediated by bio-technologies. Titmuss therefore argued that in modern societies giving has a different emphasis to do with both self-care and "... care of strangers" (1970: 212):

> In not asking for or expecting any payment of money these donors signified their belief in the willingness of other men to act altruistically in the future, and to combine together to make a gift freely available should they have a need for it ... ... As individuals they were, it may be said, taking part in the creation of a greater good transcending the good of self-love. To 'love' themselves they recognised the need to love strangers (Titmuss, 1970: 239).

Titmuss's argument therefore points out a contradiction. Gift is crucial to the wellbeing of the individual and society. But such giving is a mixture of self-love and love of others. Such ambiguity has been acknowledged by Beck and Beck-Gernsheim when they wrote about sexual relationships in late modernity: "Out of the struggle with this dilemma between love and freedom a new ethics will emerge about the importance of individuation and obligation to others. No one has the answer as to how this will work" (Beck & Beck-Gernsheim, 2002: 212). This "... altruistic individualism" as they called it (Beck & Beck-Gernsheim, 2002: 212) signifies a tension between altruism and individualisation for the self in late modernity. Beck and Beck-Gernsheim admit that the idea of 'altruistic individualism' is poorly articulated and that there is scope for "... a lot of dilemmas and paradoxes" (Beck & Beck-Gernsheim, 2002: 212). Public health governance provides some examples of such problems, in particular, the self-protecting and partner-protecting rationalities articulated with knowledge of HIV antibody serostatus.

This notion of a reciprocal but abstract altruism, in part disrupted by internal paradox, is further complicated by rationalities of disease control that spring from the idea of contagion. Contagion implies an illness or danger that spreads from person to person, such as the example of hepatitis in the blood supply. In social responses to the threat of contagion, individuals are expected to act to inhibit the spread of infection. In addition, the metaphorical city threatened by contagion, provides a way of thinking about the individual and their obligation to society. The city facing plague has many references in history, literature and social theory. For example, Foucault was interested in the idea of the city dealing with plague. In *Discipline and Punish*, he introduced Chapter 3 with a description of 17th century practices of quarantine (1982: 195–198). The management of the city and its population was focused on identifying people who had the plague (and who had not) and through controlling them, halting the spread of the epidemic. Foucault made the general point that the practices of disciplinary society incorporate traces of social responses to plague (1982: 198). Cordon sanitaire in HIV prevention could be taken as an example. He also made the point that end-of-plague festivals, like Mardi Gras, are the reverse of quarantine:

> A whole literary fiction of the festival grew up around the plague: suspended laws, lifting prohibitions, the frenzy of passing time, bodies mingling together without respect, individuals unmasked, abandoning their statutory identity and the figure under which they had been recognised, allowing a quite different truth to appear (1982: 197).

Therefore, the 'letting go' of the regulations needed for containing the plague provides a significant clue for understanding what public health governance has to achieve to control contagion. It also resonates rather strongly with the imagery of technosexuals running amok.

Plainly, plague is no longer a central problem in public health, due in part to changes in bio-technology. But, it appears that contagion has informed the practice of public health into the modern period. In addition, sexual practice appears to have special status in this arrangement.

Addressing contagion and sexual health, Pamela Cox has conducted research regarding the United Kingdom lock hospitals used in the 19th and 20th centuries to control syphilis (2007). Lock hospitals were, as their name suggests, places were sick people were involuntarily incarcerated. Cox's main argument was that the British approach to the problem of sexual health care was overtly based on voluntarism. In this regard, late 19th century and early 20th century approaches to syphilis reflected the contemporary stewardship approach to public health. However, Cox argued that such approaches incorporated a, sometimes authorised, but most often informal and therefore hidden, strategy of compulsion for some groups of people. Such groups were typically already under direct control, for example soldiers and 'fallen women'. The British approach resisted universally coercive measures for the control of syphilis because it was assumed that people should abstain from sex if they were infected, and should not ordinarily have multiple sexual partners in any case. To act to control syphilis as a matter of public policy would open government to accusations of both acknowledging and enabling vice. But this system only worked to control syphilis if those most likely to have syphilis were informally subject to direct control. Cox put it this way:

> ... this voluntary system was dependent on the fact that certain categories of people continued to be subject to unquestioned non-voluntary treatments – old style sources of contagion (soldiers and sexually transgressive women) and newly styled victims (babies and children) (Cox, 2007: 115).

In this approach to disease control, the sequestration of those with disease is achieved without compromising the overt voluntarism of public policy. In this way a seemingly archaic method of disease control can be extended into the modern period for as long as necessary.

Public health governance also appears to have a tendency to address social actors according to its own ontology of contagion. Addressing contagion, but with reference to HIV and sexual citizenship, Gayatri Reddy has conducted ethnographic research with the hijra and kothi in Hyderabad (2005). Hijras are biological men who have had their genitals removed. Kothis are in the main homosexually active men. Hijras have a liminal status in the sexual cultures of India. They are abject and disparaged but potently transgressive. However, public health approaches the Hijra according to its own rationality of the control of contagion. In this view, the epidemiological categories of Men who have

Sex with Men (MSM) and also sex worker, become the representational categories for such people. For Reddy, MSM is: "... a complex category that repudiates cultural difference in favour of a 'risk-behaviour' model" (Reddy, 2005: 265). Such categorisation of sexual identity is derived from a public health logic of contagion and is imposed on the hijra in a way that ignores how they see themselves and relate to others in society. Reddy's account gives the impression that public health is occupied with a form of self-address in the sense that it conceives of individuals and groups in terms of its own ontology of contagion.

A further complexity for public health is bio-technological innovation itself. For example, Titmuss explored the impact of the threat of hepatitis, but because of the period in which he conducted his work, he was not able to fully appraise the implications of self-knowledge of hepatitis infection for one's status in the gift economy of the blood supply. As Virginia Berridge has pointed out in relation to the blood supply in the United Kingdom, simple notions of altruism have been radically altered by technological and social changes (1997). Two factors are relevant here. In the 1980s, the United Kingdom struggled to achieve self-sufficiency in the provision of blood products. Technological developments also meant that blood products could be imported from the United States and other countries. Berridge therefore revealed that commercial markets for blood products were created in the United Kingdom, making the Titmuss model of altruism less salient. With reference to lock hospitals, Cox has pointed out how changes in the capacity to treat syphilis altered how public health approached its control (2007). In particular, the invention of antibiotics led to the separation of incarceration and bio-technological interventions and ultimately to a bio-technological control of disease. The invention of antibiotics removed the need for lock hospitals and therefore dissolved the division of free citizens and incarcerated citizens in relation to the control of syphilis. Cox therefore revealed how the relationship between bio-technology, sexually transmitted infections and the autonomy of the individual has a longstanding history. In this way technology itself becomes the way contagion rationality is mediated, which helps explain why there has been so much attention paid to HIV bio-technologies, treatment optimism and other forms of technosexuality.

Waldby and colleagues have addressed bio-technological innovation in connection with blood donation (2004). They examined contemporary perceptions of blood donation in a group of Australians donating and receiving blood and among people infected with hepatitis. Waldby and colleagues were interested to explore the relevance of notions of blood as gift in light of the theories of Mauss and Titmuss, for instance: "... altruistic citizenship identity" (2004: 1464). Waldby and colleagues found that some interviewees did see blood as a gift of part of the self, reflecting elements of Mauss's theory. They also recognised that donation could bolster social solidarity, in line with Titmuss's articulation of altruism. But Waldby and colleagues made the point that, in general, blood is so transformed by bio-technologies that it becomes like any kind of treatment available to the public. The blood products available to those who need it are no longer linked with an individual. Further, individuals who donate blood are interested in the notion that their own blood is pure and without infections. Conversely, those who cannot donate are aware that their blood is something that has to be kept away from others. Ironically, Waldby and colleagues found that individuals who donate blood were also concerned about the purity of the donated blood supply. Although they donated, some reported that it was prudent to avoid using donated blood. In this regard, such donors saw value in 'autologous' blood banking where individuals build up a personal supply of blood for their own use.

Also addressing blood donation in the Australian context, Kylie Valentine concurred with Waldby and colleagues, but made an important connection between the reconfiguration of altruism in blood donation and the public/private dimension of sexual citizenship (2005). In Australia, several categories of person are not permitted to give blood, for example, gay men, people who have injected illicit drugs, and people who may have been exposed to variant Creutzfeldt-Jakob disease (vCJD). According to Valentine: "Blood donation has become a strictly defined and finite public sphere which promises an identity of altruism and belonging to those who participate" (2005: 116). However, through bio-technologies and the knowledge they provide of infections such as HIV and hepatitis, blood donation now brings the sexual and drug using practices of individuals into blood donation and therefore into the public domain. Like public health addressing sexually transmitted infections, blood donation raises questions of model citizenship and the exclusion of errant citizens according to their sexual and drug-taking practices revealed through bio-technologies. According to Valentine, even those who can donate have a lingering anxiety concerning their potential exclusion from giving blood. There is then in modern forms of blood donation a threat of a fall from grace that applies to everyone. But, importantly, this imperilled self is defined according to bio-technologies put to the work of contagion control.

Altruism

The economics of gift that inform public health has bifurcated into a duty to give or withhold depending on one's bio-technological identity. Superficially, altruism mobilises *giving* blood. But altruism informed by contagion and articulated with bio-technological knowledge of the body figures in the *with-holding* of contaminated blood. Importantly this bifurcation is not possible without bio-technologies that can be used to identify the presence of infectious disease. Bio-technologies therefore assure that the logic of contagion is fused into the gift economy. As I have pointed out in the previous chapter, altruism has been associated with HIV prevention. I noted however that altruism has different meanings depending on HIV serostatus, for example: self-protecting is associated with people who are HIV negative and partner-protecting with those who are HIV positive. It seems that in some quarters, it is assumed that one has different responsibilities depending on one's HIV serostatus and that this is a simple system of complementary responsibilities. However, it may be that such complementary social relations are not easily exercised.

Some forms of public health appear to require altruism on the part of people with HIV. For example, several analysts have written that prevention should build on the "altruism" of HIV positive people (King-Spooner, 1999: 141). A researcher noted that: "... it is also necessary to develop prevention strategies for people with HIV infection who experience difficulty protecting their partners" (Kalichman et al., 1997: 447). A review paper recommended strategies to: "... promote norms of responsibility and protection of others in sexual matters" and "... foster the perception that HIV is still a life-threatening disease despite medical advances in treating it" (Marks et al., 1999: 303). There is a kind of symbolic violence in the idea that HIV should be portrayed as life-threatening to counteract any tendency for treatment optimism to erode commitment to safer sex. For the purposes of HIV prevention, people with HIV are expected to negate the hopes that mobilise the value of bio-technology in the management of HIV. The US Centres for Disease Control put altruism at the centre of their HIV prevention approach (Janssen et al., 2001). In this approach, a serostatus hierarchy is used to structure intervention strategy. For example, the programme is explained in this way:

> At a time of increasing risk behaviour in some communities with high HIV prevalence and among an increasing number of individuals

with HIV infection, SAFE strategies for HIV-infected individuals represent a logical evolution of prevention in an era of improved treatment. Such an approach couples a traditional infectious disease control focus on the infected person with behavioural interventions that have become standard elements in HIV prevention programmes. In this new era, for individual as well as public health reasons, every person with HIV should be voluntarily diagnosed, evaluated medically, treated according to state-of-the-art guidelines, and provided appropriate prevention services (Janssen et al., 2001: 1023).

This method follows a public health approach of directing action at the source of disease. A United States multi-city campaign was called 'HIV stops with me: prevention for positives marketing campaign' (see: *hivstopswithme.org* accessed 10 August 2008). The campaign used a mix of peer education, information materials and personal testimonials to increase self-efficacy, reduce stigma and promote safer sex among people with HIV. The underlying strategy of the campaign was the containment of the epidemic by bolstering responsible and altruistic action on the part of individuals with HIV.

This reliance on the idea of altruism on the part of people with HIV is not new. Berridge has pointed out that the United Kingdom blood supply was protected, for a time, by asking gay men to opt themselves out of donation (Berridge, 1997). Small analysed governmental responses to panic about the discovery of HIV positive health-care workers in the United Kingdom health system (Small, 1996). Small described how policy was based on a form of 'required altruism', where HIV positive health-care workers had to absent themselves from medical situations and practices that might have transmitted HIV. A policy of altruism was seen as more humane than coercive (and impractical) detection and banishment. Small showed how altruism also had the virtue of defending medicine. Altruism had the benefit of making the individual health-care worker personally responsible. To fail to act responsibly was not a failure of medical institutions or the practice of medicine in general, but of the individual practitioner. Following Small's analysis, altruism makes each person with HIV singularly responsible for managing the risks of HIV.

However, prevention altruism has some clear drawbacks. For example, Small noted how a policy of compulsory altruism on the part of HIV positive health-care workers may have discouraged openness about serostatus identity (1996). Another complexity for prevention altruism concerns gender and the labour of safer sex. Research with women with HIV concerning safer sex has explored unequal power in sexual relationships and the 'feminisation' of responsibility for condom use (Crawford et al., 1997; Lawless et al., 1996). The research also referred to the difficulties faced by women in exercising control over their own bodies without having to take on complete responsibility for contraception and safer sex. Feminisation of the work of safer sex also reflects the gendering of sexual meanings, where male sexuality, or more specifically, the male body in sex, is constructed as beyond rational control (Connell & Dowsett, 1999). Altruism therefore sits awkwardly with the construction of gender relations and the male sexual body.

Another problem for altruism is 'sero-inequality' and implications for the practice of safer sex. As I have noted in Chapter 4, different assumptions appear to be applied to sexual action depending on HIV serostatus. The notions of 'self-protection' and 'partner-protection' are the starkest examples. But it is the case that a majority of gay men report that they expect their HIV positive partners to inform them of their serostatus (Reid et al., 2002). HIV positive people have been shown to understand that they have a duty to protect the health of sexual partners, but that there were social risks to themselves in relation to disclosure of HIV status (Green & Sobo, 2000). In qualitative interviews, gay men with HIV have subscribed to the notion that they do have responsibilities to their partners (Davis, 2002). However, failure to carry out safer sex was also regarded as an act of self-destruction, suggesting the moral loading implicit in altruistic and self-protective practice. In some circumstances, people with HIV may need to act in a self-protecting manner, for instance, in relation to the impact of sexually transmitted infections on their immune system (Weatherburn et al., 1999). In this view, self-protection is relevant also for people with HIV, a perspective that exposes the HIV avoidance rationality that underpins some forms of HIV prevention. As I have noted, some gay men appear to use the internet to select sexual partners of the same HIV serostatus. Some public health practitioners are advocating that people make their HIV serostatus explicit in their online communication. Although it can be argued that serosorting and related practices are not new, the formalisation of them as matters of public policy does sit at odds with the history of safer sex. In its original form, safer sex was said to address everyone equally (Flowers, 2001). This rationality created an approach to risk management that was inclusive of HIV positive, HIV negative and untested people. This form of rationality comprised a joint effort connected with the sharing of knowledge of prevention methods such as condoms. The new bio-technologically informed government of HIV prevention divides people according to their HIV serostatus. In comparison with the old form of safer sex, the new multifarious one is a challenge for affected communities and public health alike. More abstractly, it may also be that the combination of self-protection with partner-protection presents a logical problem. If altruism is regarded as the minimal universal of safer sex, by logic it is not rational to act in self-protection. To do so would be to recognise the other as an errant citizen. Put another way, in a universe of altruistic sexual action, an act of self-protection calls into question the moral carriage of the sexual partner. A similar dynamic has been observed in relation to condom use with regular partners of HIV positive people, where condom use is seen as a disavowal of trust and intimacy (Cusick & Rhodes, 2000; Rhodes & Cusick, 2000). These effects may mean that altruism and self-protection undermine one another, or at least can lead to confusions concerning identities, intentions and responsibilities. The self-defeating logic of altruism and self-protection in relation with one another points to a major dilemma for public health wedded to such strategies of disease control.

In this light, the relational ethics of technosexual citizenship, that draws on feminism, sexual citizenship studies, and sexual health as social justice, takes on virtue as a basis for HIV prevention. Support for this position can be derived from empirical research that has used citizenship to address the sexual relations of people with HIV (Squire, 1999), heterosexual people (Bryant, 2006) and gay men (Brown, 2006). Such research shows that, reciprocity, although not symmetrical, is required to pursue sexual health and HIV prevention. In addition, relational ethics makes it possible to recognise sexual agents performing citizenship as a matter of joint action, and not identity politics (Squire, 1999). In research with gay men with HIV regarding HIV prevention, I have argued that their sexual practice was informed by a notion of cooperation (Davis, 2008). A form of adapted altruism was important to HIV prevention for gay men with HIV. In particular, interviewees acknowledged that responsibilities might differ according to HIV serostatus, but effective HIV prevention depended on cooperative action that shared moral labour and embraced both acting for the good of the other and the voluntary action of the sexual partner. These ideas concerning responsibilities combined to provide the basis for a care of the 'we' that included the mitigation of blame.

It is also plain that there is much work to be done to assist people to incorporate, or more appropriately adapt, these notions of altruism and self-protection into their sexual health care. Fortunately, public health practitioners and HIV advocacy organisations have gone some way incorporating prevention altruism into the social justice approach to sexual health. Significantly this work arises from groups advocating for people with HIV. Public health practitioners have argued that sexual health for people with HIV across the globe needs to be defined in terms of pleasurable and safe sexual experiences free from coercion, discrimination and violence (Shapiro & Ray, 2007). The National Association of People with AIDS (NAPWA) in the United States has formulated a set of guidelines for effective prevention among people with HIV (see: *napwa.org* accessed 10 August 2008). In particular, the NAPWA guidance places emphasis on the autonomy of people with HIV and the need for cooperation as the basis for effective HIV prevention. As such, the guidelines reflect how people with HIV organise collective resistance to unwelcome categorisation and the reduction of autonomy (Herdt, 2001; Parker & Aggleton, 2003). Through the sharing of responsibility in sexual partnering, the guidelines also recognise how collective and individual action can be combined in HIV prevention work. In addition, the guidelines define sexual health in terms of the capacity of people with HIV to be able to articulate their needs and act on them. In the United Kingdom and Australia, HIV prevention frameworks have similarly emphasised the autonomy of people with HIV (Triffitt & People Living With HIV/AIDS NSW, 2004; Ward, 2001).

Risk and its forensic turning

Risk is the final conceptual underpinning of public health I want to address. Risk is a concept that has come to dominate health governance, not least in the area of public health (Lupton, 1999b). Alan Petersen has written of risk discourse as "... a subtle form of individualism that involves everyone in the task of tracking down and controlling or eliminating sources of risk from their lives" (1996: 45). Risk sits in contrast with the notions of the gift economy or altruism, which arise out of functionalism. Risk draws on notions of social action that emphasise self-regulation. It could be argued that part of the schizoid quality of modern public health in general can be attributed to the ways in which it attempts to draw on modern and late modern paradigms of self and society. Notions of risk have been referred to in passing at several points in the previous discussion, for example in connection with research concerning young people who use the internet and their increased risk of being infected with sexually transmitted infections, and Viagra use or HIV bio-technologies in relation to the risk of HIV transmission among gay men. In this section, I want to focus on the contribution of the concept of risk to public health action with reference to sexually transmitted infections and HIV. In particular, I want to consider the forensic, and therefore blaming, dimension of risk culture I introduced in the previous chapter.

Ulrich Beck established the notion of the so-called risk society (see for example, Beck, 1992; Beck & Beck-Gernsheim, 2002). Risk society relies on several interconnected ideas to do with: late modern economic systems; the industrial production of risks; and a particular approach to 'individualisation'. Beck argued that late modernity has moved away from straightforward capitalism and the competition for resources. For some of us, late modernity is a time of plenty or even excess. In addition, industrial activity has created new risks. The science and technology that underpins affluence is a source of threat to the ecosystem and our own health and wellbeing, for example, pollution, industrial accidents, global warming. Because of this combination of wealth and post-industrial risks, the relationship between the individual and society has little to do with the distribution of resources, and much to do with the distribution of risks. In addition, society is now organised around the idea of the entrepreneurial individual, an assumption that informs government, social services and personal experience. Beck and Beck-Gernsheim have suggested that: "Now health, too, is not so much a gift from God as a task and achievement of the responsible citizen, who must protect and look after it or face the consequences" (2002: 139). Risk society produces forms of social exclusion through processes of individualisation:

> ... exclusion can only be properly understood against the background of individualisation or to be more precise, atomisation. It creates institutional circumstances under which individuals are cut off from traditional securities, while at the same time losing access to the basic rights and resources of modernity (2002: 207).

Beck and Beck-Gernsheim refer to this situation as "... precarious freedoms" to capture the dual effect of the unfettering of the agency of the individual and the intensification of the personalisation of risk (2002: 1). Trust and security are also implicated in risk society. According to Giddens, the late modern social actor is said to rely on, and therefore place trust in, knowledge that is dis-embedded from personal experience. Technosexual practices such as internet-mediated serosorting reflect a reliance on abstract systems. They rely on the expert knowledge systems of HIV bio-technologies that give rise to forms of HIV embodiment figured around antibody serostatus, but they are also carried out by apparently self-aware individuals.

Not all commentators have been prepared to accept risk society on face value. For Petersen, risk and its expression in public health needs to be much more thoroughly interrogated:

> Critical reflection upon the values of entrepreneurialism, consumerism, and scientism should be a part of the process of creating a more democratic society and culture. The enterprise of health promotion, however, can be seen to either take these values for granted, or reinforce them through the emphasis on individual-as-enterprise, the commodification of the body, and the reliance on expert systems (1996: 55).

Deborah Lupton has argued that risk society is a "eurocentric" concept (2002b: 333). In qualitative interviews with Australians, Lupton and Tulloch (2002a) found support for the idea that individuals recognised that they needed to take on risk as a necessary aspect of the entrepreneurial management of the life course. They therefore saw risk-taking as individualised. But the interviewees also recognised that risk was in part produced by institutions, such as commercial organisations and government. In addition, while the interviewees recognised the need to avoid risks, they also talked about it as a method of self-improvement, where, successfully dealing with risk reinforced the sense of the personal agency of the individual. Lisa Adkins has also questioned the risk society thesis in relation to a discussion of HIV antibody testing. For her it is not so much that late modernity has become risk society, but that risk is a method of organising late modernity:

> ... the techniques and practices of risk self-management, that is the techniques of self-reflexivity (such as those made available by the technology of testing) are constitutive of a social ordered in terms of categories and hierarchies of risk themselves, that is, to make up risk culture (2002: 121).

Without making reference to Beck or Giddens, Rose has offered yet another critique of risk society. In a discussion of the public health implications of genetic science, Rose regarded risk discourse as a 'technology' of government (2001). For Rose, risk thinking is central to what he referred to as bio-politics and the regulation of individuals via their own reflections on the ethics of their conduct. Risk science, such as that employed by epidemiology, helps describe where individuals fit into society in terms of their potential to develop diseases. Surveys can be used to assess the overall levels of risk in populations. Such information can help identify and manage high-risk groups and/or assist the direct management of risky individuals. Risk provides a method for informing citizens, making them active partners in public health. Rose referred to the Foucauldian concept of pastoral power to show how risk culture is both individualising and collectivising, mixes coercion and consent, and uses shame and guilt as the means of producing self-governance. Influencing how individuals reflect on the ethics of how they act on risk provides the means by which public health governance is achieved:

... the ethos of human existence – the sentiments, moral nature or guiding beliefs of persons, groups, or institutions – have come to provide the 'medium' within which the self-government of the autonomous individual can be connected up with the imperatives of good government (Rose, 2001: 18).

In relation to his argument concerning bio-politics and what he refers to as 'somatic citizenship', Rose also made the point that health is now understood in terms of rights. According to Rose, the optimally healthy body is the new universal human value. Violation of this normative, healthy body therefore becomes a transgression of human rights. This perspective partly explains the forensic turning related to HIV prevention I noted in the previous chapter. Infection of the body is now classed as one of the transgressions on this foundational right of the somatic citizen. Rose's conceptualisation of risk suggests that the tension between sexual health as absence of disease and sexual health as social justice is collapsing on a forensic turning in sexual health interventions, that is, organising citizens in terms of their contribution to sexual health problems. Lupton has made a similar point in her analysis of study of AIDS news reporting over the 1990s in Australia (1999a). For instance:

The distinction between the innocent and guilty person with HIV/AIDS was linked not so much to the source of their infection, but to the extent to which an individual with HIV/AIDS was judged to pose a risk of infection to others (1999a: 49).

As noted in the previous chapter, Douglas has discussed the forensic effects of risk culture in general (1992). Douglas argued that while risk is most often couched in terms of prediction, it also supplies the means for working backwards to determine the source of risk. A crucial concept is therefore being able to distinguish the difference between 'at risk' and 'a risk'.

With reference to HIV antibody testing, Adkins has argued that one of the forensic uses of risk is to reinforce social difference (2002). According to Adkins, HIV testing among low risk heterosexual people is widespread and growing. Such a situation sits at odds with the idea of a rational project of self-management. This is because risk rationality would suggest that low risk individuals would not make themselves available for HIV testing. Adkins argued that HIV testing for a likely HIV negative result is attractive because it reinforces one's identity as low risk and by implication as heterosexual. In this regard, Adkins's research is reminiscent of that of Waldby and colleagues and Valentine already discussed, who argued that blood donors enjoyed the idea that being able to donate blood reinforced their identities as pure sources of blood. Similarly, public health messages concerning HIV have been interpreted to refer to a risk averse "... model citizen" (Davis, 2002: 292).

It also appears to be the case that forms of technosexuality are being applied to forensic purposes. In general, technologies can assist forensic inquiry. DNA technologies can be used to determine the origin of semen, thereby facilitating the attribution of blame in sex crimes, as popularised in crime television such as *CSI* (Crime Scene Investigation) (Moore & Durkin, 2006). The internet can also be exploited in this way, or so some would have us believe. Online dating profiles, weblogs and other internet-based forms of communication are being collected and appraised for evidence of the actions of culpable citizens. In this regard, the online profiles of people who refer to themselves as barebackers have come under scrutiny. Such uses of the internet underline my point that it provides a method for making people visible under public health governance. As I have noted in Chapter 3, epidemiological studies have shown that in general, gay men who use the internet for sexual purposes are no more likely to have sex with their internet partners that might transmit HIV or other sexually transmitted infections (Elford, 2006). Although acknowledging that there is little evidence for a causal link between advertising for risky sex and actually doing it (Tewksbury, 2003), researchers have analysed the online profiles of people who espouse barebacking in an effort to develop "... a profile" of such people (Tewksbury, 2006: 379). Others suggest that the so called "... online barebacking phenomena" arises because some websites, overtly or otherwise, promote the idea that safer sex is a personal choice (Grov, 2006:

995). Some argue that barebacking is produced by internet-mediated partnering (Gauthier & Forsyth, 1999) or that particular websites encourage it (Carballo-Dieguez et al., 2006). Others argue that the dehumanising qualities of new communication technologies contribute to the desire for bareback sex (Holmes et al., 2006). Apparently, the loneliness of the cyber-age compels people to find intimacy in sex without condoms. In addition, the online mediation of barebacking discourse is itself seen as an epidemic, because of the dangerous 'exchange' of such discourses (Grov, 2004). Research such as this points to an understanding of communication technologies as sources of contagion (Lupton, 1995). The interrogation of online profiles has also undergone some refinement through distinguishing between barebackers, 'gift givers', and 'bug chasers' (Moskowitz & Roloff, 2007). Barebackers are found to use harm reduction strategies in relation to anal sex without condoms in an effort to moderate the risk of HIV transmission. Gift givers and bug chasers are recognised to seek out HIV transmission. This distinction represents a gradual focussing on errant citizens. However, not all researchers have interpreted online barebacking texts as evidence of culpable technosexual citizenship. Dowsett and colleagues have asserted that websites for same sex attracted men, including those that advocate bareback sex, exhibit ethical standards, for example: "... the overriding texture of the sites was one of an emphasis on responsibility and reciprocity" (Dowsett et al., 2008: 131). This perspective accords with the cyber-ethnographies of sexual and intimate and online life I discussed in Chapter 2. Michael Graydon has pointed out that the so-called practice of barebacking existed prior to the internet and HIV treatment (2007). In an analysis of online internet newsgroups, Graydon made note of the ways in which online communication regarding barebacking, and specifically gift giving, played with gift economy discourse. Graydon argued that this online communication is a kind of technosexual citizenship that refuses imperative. Graydon also pointed out that analyses of online communication materials are limited in terms of explaining offline sexual interaction.

Despite potential problems with the forensic research approach, it does make an important contribution to my argument. It reveals the investment of forms of public health in certain kinds of citizens and sexual relations. As I have noted in Chapter 2, the history of sexual citizenship has been marked by some key legislative moments that have impinged on the government of sexuality. The Wolfenden Inquiry and the more recent revisions of legislation concerning sexual offences in the United Kingdom have been important to the social and legal acceptance of homosexuality but also a deepening of negative sanctions on supposedly unacceptable sexual practice outside the domestic sphere (McGhee, 2004). In light of the application of risk forensics to the ordering of healthy technosexuality, it can be argued that some forms of public health are implicated in the (re)making of technosexual citizenship in terms of their own visions of the proper government of risk and risk identities. The notion that e-daters should provide information regarding their sexual health status, referring as it does to clean/unclean subjects in risk discourse (Waldby et al., 1993), is an example of interventions that subscribe to this forensic turning in the management of risk and risk subjects.

Conclusion

As I noted in Chapter 1, public health governance is complex and diverse, encompassing as it does, intervention activities, forms of knowledge, and institutions (Petersen & Lupton, 1996). Public health can be considered a total society form of governance that addresses the control of disease through the practices of individuals. But as we have seen there are various ways of addressing such practices, at least for the case of technosexuality, sexually transmitted infections, and HIV. The imperatives of gift, altruism, risk reflexivity and forensics all feature in public health governance attending to sexual health. Public health governance is also influenced by, and engaged with, bio- and communication technologies that impinge on sexually transmitted infections and HIV. Bio-technology in particular appears to be an increasingly significant aspect of public health imperatives, with subjects now divided according to the social implications of their biological characteristics. In this way, the imperatives of public health articulate with technological innovations, with implications for technosexual citizenship. Because bio-technologies change so rapidly, the implications for public health imperatives also alter rapidly.

Despite (or perhaps because of) being open to change, public health governance is like a Colossus of social theory, with one foot in modern, and one foot in late modern, notions of self and society. Public health also seeks to encompass an immense range of intervention activities, forms of knowledge, and institutions. Some of these assumptions derive from functionalist notions of altruism mixed with the rationality of contagion control. Others embrace late modern notions of self-determining, risk averse subjects. There have been calls for compliance policies and the regulation of e-dating websites. Some have argued that people should make their sexual health histories visible in their internet communication, not as a matter of voluntary action or in terms of moderating discrimination, but as part of a policy of disease control. Such public health appears to rely on constraining the action of individuals by encouraging the shaping of online social environments so that they work to prevent sexually transmitted infections and HIV. In addition, some social science has bent itself to a kind of forensic inquiry, tracing out the lines of transgression and culpability in the products of internet-based sexuality, and unwittingly or not, entering into the politics of blame. Public health practitioners have also called for altruism on the part of people with HIV and by extension, those who know they have other sexually transmitted infections. In this view, individuals who know they have an infection have a duty to others. This form of public health governance appeals to social obligation through notions of altruism, particularly by asking people who know they have an infection of some kind to be careful not to infect others. But public health also advocates self-protection. This imperative relies on notions of calculating, risk averse individuals, acting to protect themselves. This rationality appears to apply to those who know or believe that they do not have an infection.

As I have shown, there may be some problems with the mixture of these imperatives for technosexual citizenship. For example, the reference to altruistic and self-protective imperatives in public health is outwardly a neat arrangement of citizens according to their biological characteristics. Public health therefore works to supply a logic for sociality that coheres with its own vision of altruism, contagion and bio-technological knowledge. But it is not clear how such subjects should relate to one another. It has long been recognised that pure altruism is, in practice, a fictional ideal. The work of Mauss, Titmuss and others has revealed that the 'love of others' and 'love of the self' are one. But some forms of public health work to prise apart love of others (altruism) and self love (self-protection). These purified imperatives satisfy a bio-technological logic of the presence or absence of sexually transmitted infections and HIV, but they may not enable social actors to negotiate their sexual inter-relations. Mauss, Titmuss and others have argued that society depends on reciprocal relations, or more abstractly, loving one another. This co-extensive love of others/love of self is a guarantee of equivalence in reciprocal relations, despite biological knowledge to the contrary. This way of addressing social obligation also forms a point of connection with the reciprocal ethics that seem to provide the basis for forms of technosexual citizenship more generally. But despite drawing on functionalist notions of altruism, some forms of public health governance eschew the equivalence implied in the ethics of reciprocity and appear to be interested in calling into being technosexual citizens typed according to those who can only love others, or themselves, but not types of technosexual citizens who can love one another. In view of these conceptual troubles, the adapted altruism advocated by community-groups for people with HIV and the notions of relational ethics for technosexual citizenship take on deep significance. These approaches are pragmatic responses to the challenge of forming social and sexual relations that reconcile obligations and autonomy in relation to the imperatives of preventing sexually transmitted infections and HIV and the knowledges and practices that arise through technological innovation. These approaches also show an awareness of the inconsistencies and clashes in public health governance.

We can recognise then that the public health governance of technosexuality is multiple, fluid, and open to contestation. It is important to note however, that public health governance is not the only way that social difference is asserted in social relations. And, of course, public health may not seem contestable from the point of view of the institutions that produce it. In addition, my examples may not characterise all public health governance. But it is important to consider how such examples can arise. It is my argument that it is the multiple character of public health imperatives articulated with technological innovations that makes these examples possible. We need to consider therefore how public health governance appears to citizens engaged with technosexuality. From their point of view, public health governance may well seem multiple and contradictory.

It is not of course possible to turn away from this situation. Following Greco and Rose noted in Chapter 1 and others who have developed a similar line of argument, we need a more thoroughly reflexive public health governance and a political engagement with its technologies. Technosexuality is a challenging preoccupation for public health precisely because of the old problem of sex, technological change and government. As Gordo-Lopez and Cleminson have argued, technological changes that mobilise desires necessarily inspire forms of social repression, thereby assuring the sexual power of technological innovation (2004). As previous chapters have demonstrated, the general shape of the public health government of technosexuality accords with this notion. Technosexual forms are seen as dangerous for public health but also the means through which public health governance can be achieved. This chapter has served to demonstrate how technologies and public health articulate in yet another way. Public health imperatives are joined with the innovations of bio-technological knowledge to derive forms of technosexual citizenship figured around the prevention of sexually transmitted infections and HIV. In the next chapter, I want to develop this notion of the articulation of technology and public health governance. As we will see, bio- and communication technologies work, severally and jointly, to help make technosexual citizens visible, supplying an important governmental strategy for public health.

6
Technological Visibilities

This chapter makes a case for I want to call technosexual visibility and its ramifications for public health governance. As I have discussed, depictions of internet-based sexuality often draw on the idea that the internet is dangerous because netizens can hide their identities. But at the same time, it is not easy to ignore how the internet makes sexuality visible in new ways. As interactive screen media, the internet is arguably a visual technology. Some have suggested that the internet is truly panoptic because it allows the collection of information regarding the behaviour of individual users (Jordan, 1999). Such perspectives are often ignored in media portrayals of the dangers of the internet. But as I will detail below, when commentators draw attention to the dangers of the internet, they necessarily rely on the visibility that the internet makes possible. The popular media also extends this visibility, by relaying these depictions into the public sphere. It will be my argument that, like media on the subject, public health governance is coming to rely on technosexuality because it provides a method for revealing individuals in relation to their sexual practices. I also want to suggest that, through this kind of engagement with technosexuality, public health governance is connected with political questions concerning acceptable sexual practice.

This notion of visibility builds on elements of previous discussions. At several points in this book I have made use of the language of visibility. In Chapter 2, I used the idea of the questing avatar to draw attention to the ways in which online game environments and other parts of the internet create opportunities for visualising the self, on occasion in relation to intimacy and sexuality. I noted that online interaction is informed by a relational ethics of authenticity and transparency. In Chapter 3 in connection with the case study of e-dating, I explored debate concerning the narcissistic aspects of internet-mediated intimate and sexual life. To some extent, the self-presentation practices of internet-based communication are like mirrors in the way that people can construct and modify images of themselves. However, technosexual visibility is not just a product of the internet. It is possible to argue that visibility is derived from the methods of public health itself. To help explain this idea I would like to use an example. I was first employed to do HIV research in the United Kingdom in a sexual health clinic. On my first day I was shown around the clinic so I could understand the different aspects of work carried out there. I was taken to the laboratory where tissue specimens from patients were taken for analysis. I was shown how slides of skin cells were prepared with chemical colour stains to reveal the presence (or not) of infections. The slides so rendered were placed under a microscope so that the presence (or not) of infection could be observed and documented. The diagnosis based on the slide of infected cells allowed the prescribing clinician to make appropriate decisions regarding treatment. I never again set foot in the laboratory, but have always remembered that moment as a revelation of the hidden interior of sexual health care. I think I was meant to be impressed by the spatial and therefore temporal proximity of walk-in sexual health services with technological and scientific procedures for the detection of the proof of infections. I was definitely struck by the way such an arrangement materialised what I take to be the central rationality of sexual health care provision following the disease model. In particular, the spatial and temporal arrangement of walk-in patients, tissue samples taken from patients, imaging technologies, and the production of proof, is a system that hinges on the observation of the biological characteristics of the individual. Through such observation, proof is available that provides the basis for effective, efficient, and ethical clinical care. These are vital objectives for public health. But I want to argue that this observational control of infectious diseases in the individual body and through it the population, is a method that is being extended through technosexuality. The orthodox view of technosexuality is that, to some extent, it challenges public health by, in some way or another, facilitating the transmission of sexually transmitted infections and HIV. But it is also possible to argue that technosexuality figured in appropriate ways, operates as a method for furthering public health governance in technologically-mediated societies.

This emphasis on visibility has an obvious association with Foucault and the medical gaze (1976). For example, drawing on Foucault, authors have pointed out how HIV bio-technologies help create forms of visibility

(Heaphy, 1996; Race, 2001). Foucault argued that medical power over health is exercised in the authority to trace the boundaries between the organs of the body and name these according to a medical language of normal and pathological embodiment. He also maintained that this strategy of bringing a medical body into existence was extended into the spatial organisation of bodies according to medical categories in clinics and hospitals and beyond. In relation to innovative health technologies, Webster has referred to Foucault's notion of the medical gaze to discuss health technologies and authority (2007). Authority over the meaning of embodied signs provides a basic form of power for medical practitioners. This power can be extended through bio-technologies. But Webster also raised a critique concerning the problem of the infinite regress of Foucauldian discourse analysis, pointing out that in such analyses: " ... there is no foundation for critique that is not itself simply another form of discourse" (Webster, 2007: 39). In this regard, he commented that some feminist scholarship has also found fault with Foucauldian discourse analysis, because it does not in the end furnish the means for a proper critique of unequal power over the body, gender relations and so on. I share these reservations, but I want to use this notion of gaze to show how visibility forms a point of continuity for internet and bio-technologies and their hybrids, and therefore explains their affinity with forms of public health governance. This kind of analysis has not been widely conducted for the specific circumstances of technosexuality and public health governance, and there are some important insights to be gained. In particular, I want to consider the idea that forms of technosexuality supply an epistemic strategy for the governance of technosexual citizens. The internet performs the epistemological function of imaging technology such as the microscope. But in place of infections, the focus is on practices that have implications for sexually transmitted infections and HIV, and through these, the ethics of sexual conduct. I am not of course arguing that the internet permits observation of sexual practices that might transmit sexually transmitted infections and HIV. But as I will argue, online profiles, chatroom discussions and other expressions of technosexuality, are attractive to public health governance because they suggest that it is possible to observe the intimate and sexual life of citizens in ways that are not otherwise available. Practices such as serosorting expressed in online communication, or so-called barebacking websites, can be taken as examples.

In the following sections, I first establish in more detail what I mean by technosexual visibility. Next, I consider how visibility finds expression in media representations of the so-called practice of barebacking among gay men and other apparent transgressions of public health advice concerning HIV. As I have done elsewhere, I will refer to these stories as 'spectacular risk' to draw attention to the double meaning of extremity and visibility (Davis, in press). I want to focus on spectacular risk to draw attention to the mediatisation of public health governance. In the final section of this chapter, I discuss the ethical questions that spectacular risk implies for technosexuality. In particular, I want to raise the debate regarding the negative effects of the unbridled individualism that is said to be axiomatic to spectacular risk.

Technology and visibility

The internet is making all manner of aspects of sexual practices visible. Cyber-ethnographies of intimate online experience have suggested that forms of self-presentation reveal social and psychological processes. In this regard the notional questing avatar is a key figure. Online life is sustained via an ethics of authenticity and transparency. E-dating practices require that people reveal themselves in terms of their desires in order to make connections with others. Researchers are observing what people do online as the basis for evaluating risk for sexually transmitted infections and HIV. The coding and categorisation capacities of internet technologies applied to the mediation of sexual practice have an affinity with biotechnologies that provide coded information concerning the sexual health status of the body. The practice of internet-mediated serosorting is an example of such affinity. Some public health practitioners are advocating as a matter of public policy, that people should represent their sexual health status in their profiles and other forms of communication. Taken together, these examples do lend support to the idea that forms of technosexuality provide an important method for observing and regulating sexual practice under public health governance.

I am not alone in making an argument along these lines. Waldby has argued that computer technologies extend the medical gaze in new and surprising ways and that such visibility is attractive to medicine because it creates a seductive illusion of superior control over the body. In this sense, the visibility produced by technosexuality is enticing for public health governance because it too exhibits the promise of more effective observation and regulation. Waldby has made this argument in connection with the Visible Human Project (VHP) (2000). The VHP is a computer based anatomy text for medical teaching hosted by the United States, National Library of Medicine (*nlm.nih.gov/research/visible/*

visible_human.html accessed 10 August 2008). The VHP uses computer technology to create three-dimensional images of the bodies of a man and a woman. These images are accessible via the internet for teaching. Apparently, different views of the bodies can be summoned at the click of a mouse. Stunningly, the bodies are actual bodies that have been sliced and scanned into a computer programme. The VHP therefore works to fuse together computer technology, the body, and the medical gaze. The way in which the images were made and their high quality, three-dimensional attributes, brings flesh and virtual very close together, creating a permanent, manipulable, cross-reference of fleshly and virtual embodiment. Waldby's discussion of the VHP addressed the power of information technologies to make the body visible for biomedical purposes with some surprising implications for how human life is understood. As Waldby put it, the VHP has technological capacities that have a deep attraction for users:

> Its limitless capacity to decompose and recompose the virtual corpse lends it to biomedical fantasising about human life, and Life in general, as an informational economy which can be animated, reproduced, written and rewritten, through biomedical management (2000: 36–37).

Waldby therefore suggested that the VHP technology is appealing because it permits the extension of a fantasy of control over the human body. Unlike a text book which offers two-dimensional images at the turn of the page, the VHP offers the illusion of three dimensional images that can be easily viewed from different standpoints. Through this more thorough-going, visual inspection of the human body, the VHP thus offers its users a sense of the perfection of the medical gaze, and therefore a new realisation of medical authority over health. This fantasy of control through visibility is also the underlying rationality of other uses of computer technology in health, such as the building of national online patient record databases (Webster, 2007). The interest of public health in technosexual visibility follows the same pattern. Referring to Braidotti, Waldby also suggested that the VHP is an:

> ... an icon of medical pornography. It is a field of visual fantasisation which plays out certain forms of mastery over a completely compliant, imaginary body, whose morphology has no integrity of its own, but is completely at the disposal of the master (2000: 37).

Waldby has therefore pointed out that such uses of computer technology are erotic in the sense that the viewer/manipulator can use the technology to express their desires, academic, voyeuristic or both. In this sense, the manipulation of the images of bodies in the VHP resembles the self-animation aspects of the avatars of online gaming. On this basis, it could be argued that the VHP itself is a form of technosexuality.

Technosexuality offers similar effects for public health governance. The internet is a form of interactive, screen media which assures its status as a method for circulating information and images. The personal nature of online images and the desires they express, gives the impression that technosexuality provides a window on sexual practice. The internet also permits the coding of selves and intentions, providing a rich source of ready-made data for research inquiry. As I have argued, the internet also permits the coding of bio-technological knowledge such as sexual health status. In the public health gaze, such coding fixes such bio-technologically identified individuals in the media, linking their sexual health status with intentions regarding sexual practices. Technosexuality also provides a communication method for research, allowing access to sexually active populations. The visual property of technosexuality and its salience for public health is also revealed in the forensic research that has analysed online profiles, as I discussed in Chapter 5. As I have also noted, some forms of public health are asking individuals to make themselves more visible by indicating their health status in their online communication (Levine & Klausner, 2005).

There is cause to argue therefore that technosexual visibility has considerable appeal for public health governance. But there is also an important difference between technosexual and other technological visibilities. Technosexual visibility contradicts the typical account of the internet that attributes its dangers to its capacity for anonymous social interaction. As I have argued, anonymity is only one aspect of the visibility that characterises technosexuality. Anonymity in an absolute sense is not technically possible given the capacities of the internet to collect information regarding individuals and their practices. I have suggested that anonymity is a mode of (non)visibility in a context where authenticity and transparency are the ethical standards of interaction that help make online social and sexual experience work as social forms. The notion that people are able to effectively hide their identities online is based on an assumption that the ontology of online life is relative to that of offline life. It assumes both that people do not hide their identities offline (or at least not so easily) and that online life is never as authentic as offline life. Both these assumptions are likely to be crudely deterministic.

Spectacular risk, ethnographic media and forensic research

Public health is attracted to technosexual visibility, not just because it reveals dangers, but because it suggests itself as a window on sexual practice and therefore the means for improved governance of the risks of sexually transmitted infections and HIV. However, this reliance on aspects of technosexual visibility attaches public health governance to an ambiguity regarding the public and private status of technosexuality and therefore questions of acceptable sexual conduct. This ambiguity and its consequences is most clearly seen in relation to the practice of so-called barebacking among gay men. As I have noted, barebacking is the idea that some gay men choose to not use condoms for anal sex. It is said that some gay men use the internet to find such bareback partners. Such internet-mediated barebacking has come into view as a public health problem through technosexual visibility. The rejection of condoms for anal sex is said to reflect a position regarding HIV bio-technologies that they reduce the transmission of the virus and its health consequences in general. The idea of barebacking is also seen as a transgression of public health advice. Weatherburn and colleagues have noted that there has been a moral panic, or as they refer to it, a "... gay sex hysteria", concerning this practice in the media and in some forms of public health research and commentary (2003: 1). Such stories and research can be taken to be examples of what Halperin has referred to as the psycho-pathologisation of the sexual practices of gay men (2007). These stories could also be regarded as a form of hetero-normative sexualisation of gay men's sexuality (Lee, 2007). It is impor-tant to note that this moral panic is not restricted to the sexual practices of gay men. Media stories surrounding court cases regarding HIV trans-mission have addressed the sexual practices of heterosexual men through a combination of racism and moral judgement (Persson & Newman, 2008). With reference to gay men however, there is a special techno-sexual inflection because barebacking media stories refer to both the internet and HIV treatment as important aspects of such practice. I use the term spectacular risk to draw attention to the quality of these depictions of internet-mediated barebacking that make it seem like a superlative transgression of acceptable sexual ethics, and through such depictions, its visibility as extreme risk (Davis, in press). As I will argue, the public/private ambiguity of technosexual visibility gives the spec-tacular risk narrative its force and resonance in mediatised societies that give emphasis to stories of intimate and sexual life. I also want to suggest that technosexual visibility and the spectacular risk narrative combine in a specific use of the ethnographic interview in popular media regarding barebacking. At the same time, social research is drawing on this spectacular risk narrative to justify itself. Such uses of technosexual visibility give rise to a new kind of spectatorship where ethnography and scandal journalism crossover in a mediatised discourse of public health governance.

We are said to live in mediatised societies where the private lives of citizens are very much public concerns. Technosexual visibility reflects this aspect of sexuality in mediatised societies. Plummer has discussed the explosion of stories regarding intimate and sexual citizenship in the popular media (Plummer, 2003). For example, the intimate and sexual lives of citizens are a prominent feature of reality television, talk shows, and gossip magazines. According to Plummer, the popular media thus transmits stories of the private sphere of intimate and sexual life into the public sphere. It supplies narratives of intimate life for individuals to consume. Plummer has suggested that the mediatisation of narratives of intimate life has become the means through which we acquire a sense of ourselves as sexual citizens. Forms of technosexuality can be taken to operate in a similar manner. Practices such as e-dating and other forms of internet-mediated sexual interaction are private in the sense that they reflect desires and aspirations and are often revealing of personal information and images. But these forms of communication are also public in the sense that they exist for others in the online world. E-dating resonates with the media in general in another way. With reference to an analysis of online profiles posted to *Match.Com*, Arvidsson has suggested how online profiles reflect the confessional/therapeutic mode of self-engagement that has found expression in television talk shows such as *Oprah* (2006).

The public/private quality of technosexual visibility intersects with a debate in sexual citizenship regarding heteronormative domesticity. In Chapter 2, I discussed McGhee's account of changes to sex offences legislation in the United Kingdom, that has given rise to the "de-homosexualisation" of such laws coupled with increased regulation of inappropriate sexual behaviour outside the domestic sphere (2004: 368). McGhee argued that this double movement has the effect of legitimising a 'normal, domesticated sexuality'. Popular media surrounding the intimate and sexual lives of citizens derives some of its frisson from this division of private/public. In systems of sexual citizenship that emphasise a division of acceptable private and unacceptable public sexual practice, technosexual visibility is troublesome because it is both private and public. As McGhee noted himself, it may become more difficult to address forms of technosexuality in creative ways if such practices are seen to sit outside appropriate, private and, above all, domesticated sexuality (2004). Technosexuality may become internally divided by, or figured around a tension between, those practices that sustain and extend notions of heteronormative domesticity and those that are seen as unacceptable. This is the argument made by some ethnographers of queer online life who have argued for the digital closet, or in other words, the idea that technosexuality offers a method for rendering as perverse, sexual interests that exist outside the domestic, heteronormative sphere (Phillips, 2002). It may be that technosexuality can only be approached by public health in terms that are consistent with its status as a troublesome or unacceptable form of sexuality.

It seems that popular media has exploited technosexual visibility precisely because of its ambiguous public/private quality and implications for acceptable conduct. Such exploitation has been achieved by drawing on the ways in which the internet makes sexuality visible and by inventing a discourse of spectacular risk for depictions of so-called barebacking among gay men. For example, one of the first articles to establish the spectacular risk narrative depicted an online chat with a man seeking sex without condoms (Signorile, 1997). The chatter was said to have not known his HIV antibody serostatus, but was unconcerned because he believed that HIV treatments reduced the negative health consequences of HIV infection. Since 1997, there have been several other such spectacular risk articles in the United States mainstream and gay men's press, for example: *Bay Area Reporter* (Beswick, 2000); and *POZ* (Gendin, 1999; Scarce, 1999). Articles have also been published in the United Kingdom, for example: *The Guardian* (Wells, 2000); *The Independent* (Elliott, 2004); *The Mail on Sunday* (Laza, 2003). The idea of transgressive risk-taking and its intersections with technosexuality is a dominant theme in these stories. However, not all writers have taken spectacular risk on face value. For example, in the United Kingdom, several authors in the gay men's press have questioned the moral panic of barebacking stories (see: Cairns, 2000; Maguire, 2000).

Despite the countervailing stories of what barebacking represents, the spectacular risk narrative has continued to be used in the media, for example, in the United States gay men's magazine, *The Advocate*, (Kennedy, 2006). A 2003 article in the *Rolling Stone* exemplified the spectacular risk narrative (Freeman, 2003: online source). This article has been much discussed in the literature (see for example: Graydon, 2007). This particular formation of the spectacular risk story had the requisite elements of transgression, internet-mediated sexual partnering and views regarding

HIV bio-technologies. It featured an interview with a gay man depicted as a 'bug chaser': someone who used the internet to locate partners for risky sex; trivialised HIV; and overestimated the effects of HIV treatment in counteracting the damaging effects of HIV infection. The story juxtaposed the banality of a meeting over coffee to conduct the interview with the spectacular rejection of public health advice.

My point here is to argue that stories such as these make a particular form of risk-taking visible, sometimes by using technosexual visibility itself as source data. There is an obvious difference between magazine stories and social science in terms of ethics and epistemology. For example, the practice of reporting on single online chats or interviews as the basis for assertions concerning the reported behaviours of so-called barebackers or bug chasers, would not stand up very well under academic peer review. It seems however that it is acceptable to publish such stories on the basis that apparent disregard for safer sex overshadows any considerations of ethics or truth-claims. This approach is a specific instance of what I refer to as technosexual visibility. The supposedly reprehensible practice of securing sexual partners for risky sex exhibited in online communication is treated as a window on the private lives of errant citizens. Indeed, the spectacular quality of these stories relies on making such intimate and sexual practices visible. In this situation, media stories draw on the visibility of internet-mediated sexual practices, in a similar manner to public health research on the subject. Spectacular risk stories can therefore be taken as a form of public health governance. They help transfer the techniques of public health to the mass media and possibly into sexual culture itself. In addition, spectacular risk stories exploit the dual private/public quality of internet-based communication. The internet puts such private aspects of life into the public domain, amenable to scrutiny and therefore available for incorporation into media stories.

Such spectacular risk stories resonate with the 'reality' crime genre of broadcast television. In their book, *Reality TV: Realism and revelation*, Biressi and Nunn have pointed out that real crime media is a fusion of drama and documentary (2005). As such, real crime media combines dramatised reconstructions, CCTV, mobile phone images, testimonials and moralising voice-overs. Like reality crime media, spectacular risk stories draw together commentary, documentary and testimonial. The internet lends itself to this spectacular risk genre because the products of cyber-culture, such as online chat, are easily collected. Such products are analogous with the CCTV and mobile phone images used in real crime media. They have a seductive 'reality' that lends ontological weight to spectacular risk stories. Assembled to focus on risk-taking, they are taken to provide windows on what is 'really' happening. In addition, the adoption of the reality genre fits well with a generalised social conservatism concerning the moral degeneracy of late modern societies, often attributed to new technologies such as the internet (Tomlinson, 1999). As I have pointed out, the forensic turning in the risk rationality of public health provides the means for assigning blame. This forensic turning is reflected in research that has interrogated barebacking websites and online communication for evidence of errant citizenship. Spectacular risk stories resonate with such a forensic turning, most obviously because they employ the methods of the real crime genre, but also because they imply blame, or at least create the conditions whereby blame can be apportioned.

Following Waldby, there is also reason to consider if spectacular risk stories are indeed a form of pornography, or at least a virtual form of transgressive sexual practice made available for general consumption. Barebacking stories have the voyeuristic qualities of popular media in general (Denzin, 1995). As with television programmes that rely on the reality genre, barebacking stories may provide a form of libidinal satisfaction for the audience (Biressi & Nunn, 2005). Readers can indulge in erotic, transgressive practice, without actually doing it. They can therefore partake in the symbolic exchange of images of sexual hedonism and the rejection of risk reduction advice. We could argue that this virtual barebacking is a form of safe sex, a virtual sublimation of the urges we may share. But there are questions therefore, of the kinds of ethics of technosexual citizenship in play, and the exploitation of the notional barebacker or bug chaser. In particular, readers of spectacular risk stories, if they so choose, can subscribe to a notion of themselves as ethically superior and pretend that barebacking is somehow restricted to the ethically defective. As Brown has argued in relation to moral panic and barebacking, spectacular risk stories help re-inscribe an oppositional system of model and errant citizens (2006).

The spectacular risk narrative may also be historically specific. In early periods of the epidemic, the knowledge that AIDS was caused by a sexually transmissible, blood-borne virus led to what was then called the AIDS crisis (Epstein, 1996). The crisis is said to have mobilised action to alert communities, such as gay men and drug-users, of the new danger and to encourage safer sex and sterile injecting drug use. One of the main reasons for such community-based action was the reluctance of government to act. Public health was unable or unwilling to engage with stigmaed sexual and drug-using practices (Watney, 2000).

In this early stage of the AIDS crisis, it was not easy to raise moral outrage over unsafe sex, although of course, such a line of argument did appear in the mainstream press (for instance, see analysis of the British press on AIDS: Beharrell, 1993). But a moral outrage over unsafe sex was not easy to articulate because gay and drug-using communities were consumed with responding to the threat of AIDS and caring for those who became ill, eking out meagre resources, and galvanising risk reduction practices. The rationality of HIV prevention concerned the encouragement of condom use and sterile injecting where they had not been the norm. Spectacular risk stories reverse this rationality to draw attention to the transgression of a normative condom use.

Spectacular risk stories may also represent a re-focusing of the practical and ethical management of the epidemic in relation to changes in the science, technology and government that underpins it. The invention of safer sex as a method and ethical stance on risk reduction was predicated on the stigma of some sexual and drug-using practices, the social status of affected communities, and the slow, reluctant action of government. It was inevitable then that as these conditions softened and reformed in new ways, assumptions regarding the ethics of safer sex would also alter. Sontag in writing about HIV and AIDS in 1988 referred to the interplay of calculability, uncertainty and the governance of the present:

> Being able to estimate how matters will evolve into the future is an inevitable by-product of a more sophisticated (quantifiable, testable) understanding of process, social as well as scientific. The ability to project events with some accuracy into the future enlarged what power consisted of, because it was a vast new source of instructions about how to deal with the present (Sontag, 1988: 89).

Sontag's account of knowledge and power helps explain how new technologies such as effective HIV treatment and the internet might be implicated in the gradual focusing of requirements on conduct. As I have pointed out, Treichler has also noted how the end of AIDS story was prefigured in various speculative accounts of the epidemic, and is, in effect, built into the crisis discourse (Treichler, 1999: 325). We can argue therefore that social, technological and governmental changes have always had a relationship with the discursive management of HIV risk and sexual practice.

Based on this argument regarding crisis discourse and the notion of gradual focusing of governance, we are led to consider if the spectacular risk narrative represents the excess of crisis finding new applications in this post-internet, post-treatment era. At least in the affluent global North, HIV infection is now regarded as a chronic, manageable illness (Green & Smith, 2004). The introduction of effective HIV treatments in the mid 1990s and other improvements in the clinical management of HIV infection have resulted in changes concerning the clinical and symbolic meaning of HIV and AIDS. Further, media analyses of HIV and AIDS stories have identified the passing of the organising discourse of crisis (Lupton, 1998). The spectacular risk genre could be regarded as a turning back to panic discourse, in a manner that reveals both an awareness of the subsiding of AIDS as 'crisis', but also an invitation to consider new dangers. In this regard, such stories reveal a 'neo-crisis' rationality applied to risk, sex and technology. But in place of urgency concerning AIDS and the mobilisation of collective action to warn, protect and care, neo-crisis discourse is bound up with outrage concerning those who are seen to be transgressing accepted sexual conduct.

The politics of technosexual transgressions

By drawing on a kind of realism of transgression made possible via techno-sexuality, spectacular risk stories further controversy regarding the ethical status of technosexual forms. These stories also have the effect of ensuring that technosexuality takes a central position in the cultural contest regarding what will count as acceptable sexual practice in technologically-mediated societies. Spectacular risk may also provide a solution for public health in relation to changes in the patterns of risk behaviour among people at risk of sexually transmitted infections and HIV. For example, researchers have begun to argue that there is cause for concern with regard to HIV transmission among gay men. Research from the United Kingdom (Dodds et al., 2004), Australia (Prestage et al., 2005) and the United States (Wolitski et al., 2001) has indicated that from 1996/7, reported risky sexual practice began to increase, suggesting that the practice of safer sex among gay men may have weakened. Attempts have been made to explain these changes, including internet-mediated partnering discussed in Chapter 3, and the advent of effective HIV treatment discussed in Chapter 4. As I have shown, none of these explanations are entirely convincing. In the face of weak explanations for these historic changes in sexual practice, researchers have resorted to the idea that changes must be determined by some combination of all these factors. This multi-factorial position is itself limited because it combines explanations that have ambiguous support at best. It is my argument that it is no surprise that the spectacular risk narrative arises in the face of increases in reported risk behaviour for which we lack a satisfactory explanation. Because the idea of bare-backing is said to reflect the volition of an autonomous sexual actor, it requires no explanation. Because it is risk-taking for risk-taking's sake, it is the source of its own proof. It is an understanding of risk behaviour that is stripped of questions regarding the fallibility of both the method of safer sex and the knowledge and skills of the individual. Despite efforts to the contrary, it is a form of risk that cannot be effectively explained in terms of psychological deficits or structural barriers. In fact, as I will discuss, any attempt at explanation of barebacking itself turns to the variables that have been applied to explanations of the general case of anal sex without condoms in previous stages of the epidemic. Through the repudiation of self and the other implicit in such risk practice, it also represents a kind of individualism in excess. Spectacular risk has the effect therefore of accentuating ethical questions regarding technosexual selves, particularly in relation to what is seen as a neo-liberal form of autonomous action that is undermining public health efforts to control sexually transmitted infections and HIV.

One of the challenges of so-called barebacking is that it is not easily defined in behavioural terms. In a review of risk behaviour research Wolitski has pointed out this problem and argued that while there is pre-existing research that does explain anal sex without condoms among gay men, there is a lack of an explanation for the notion that some gay men appear to 'consciously' reject safer sex (2007). I have noted already that Douglas has addressed the concern that people might choose to take risks (1992). For Douglas, such choices are not explainable as a matter of psychology or sociology, because they reflect membership of groups constituted in risk culture. Nevertheless, Wolitski provided a map of six factors that appear to be contributing to 'barebacking', some of which are recognisable as dimensions of technosexuality: the advent of effective HIV treatment; complex decision-making regarding HIV antibody serostatus and bio-technologies; the advent of internet-based sexual networking; illicit drug use in and around sexual intercourse; safer sex fatigue; and changes in the scope and content of public health approaches. The problem with these explanations is that they also apply to anal sex without condoms in general. Wolitski also noted that researchers do not always agree on how to define barebacking. Likewise, it appears that gay men do not always share the definitions of barebacking used by researchers. Huebner and colleagues asked gay men to categorise various risky sexual scenarios with terms including 'barebacking' (2006). The respondents were found to refer to any anal sex without condoms as barebacking, that is, regardless of the intentions of the actors. Research participants are not alone in making this slippage from barebacking as intentional risky sex to any risky sexual practice. In other research, ostensibly exploring barebacking among gay men, Suarez and colleagues enumerated the various social and psychological contexts of all anal sex without condoms (2001). This research suggests that the scrutiny of barebacking leads back to the general case of the conditions of anal sex without condoms. In another example, researchers have linked barebacking to the cultural significance of the exchange of semen (Holmes & Warner, 2005). This notion has been discussed in previous research in relation to anal sex in general (Flowers et al., 1997). Likewise, psychotherapists working with gay men have attributed barebacking to psychosocial factors that, arguably, have been linked with anal sex without condoms in general for some time (Cole, 2007; Shernoff, 2006). As Michael Hurley has noted in connection with the recent rise in reported risky behaviour among gay men in Australia: "... there is no set of definitive reasons why the increase should be understood as having intrinsically different causes than those involved in ongoing infections over the last decade" (2003: 5). We could argue therefore that spectacular risk narrative has sponsored its own research culture that may not be useful in terms of advancing knowledge.

Some researchers have addressed barebacking as transgression, somewhat furthering the spectacular risk narrative. However, others have questioned whether barebacking is transgression in any case. Michelle Crossley has argued that because homosexuality is a transgression of heteronormativity and that such transgression is a reflection of the psyches of gay men, transgression of public health guidelines is unconscious (2004). This notion of unconscious resistance of heteronormativity through a resistance of public health governance is faulty because it elides heteronormativity and the good governance of health, essentialises gay identity, and leaves no room for an explanation of transgression on the part of heterosexual people (Flowers & Langdridge, 2007). It also appears to subscribe to, and therefore reinforce, spectacular risk narrative. In contrast, Damien Riggs has argued that because barebacking discourse reinforces the sanctioned status of adherence to public health guidelines and therefore actually reinforces heteronormativity, it cannot be properly understood as transgressive (2006). Riggs argued that the outrage over barebacking provides a method for transferring the heterosex=good and homosex=bad duality to safer sex and barebacking, respectively. Riggs also suggested that this duality of good sex/bad sex compels practices such as serosorting. Under 'hetero-normative' governance of good sexual health, gay men are encouraged to find forms of sexual interaction that are not open to judgements of 'bad sex'. In this regard, Riggs's analysis is reminiscent of that of Brown's regarding the model/errant citizen opposition in his account of bare-backing panic in Seattle (2006). Part of the reason for panic was that public health officials were predicting a rise in new infections based on the information that was available to them concerning the increase in reported sex without condoms among gay men. As time went on, it became clear that the expected increase in HIV transmission did not transpire. As Brown observed, gay men and public health officials were: " ... struggling over imperfect, situated knowledge while all agonistically performing political obligation in contested ways" (Brown, 2006: 885). He noted how the spectacular risk narrative fixed on a notional, errant, technosexual citizen and, on that basis, provided an alibi for public health struggling with new challenges, some of which did not come into being. Spectacular risk also served the agenda of some members of the gay community who wanted to argue that some gay men were irresponsible and to blame for a continuing epidemic.

This politics of transgression expressed through spectacular risk is reflected in a debate concerning individualism in HIV prevention. Some have argued that a form of neo-liberal individualism promoted by public health attending to the risk-averse social actor undermines inter-ventions because it breaks down social obligation. For example, it is said that the dominant forms of public health intervention regarding HIV speak to an individualised subject and therefore may imply indi-vidualistic action in the negotiation of safer sex (Dodds, 2002). As Dodds argued, an analysis of HIV prevention materials revealed that they mainly addressed individual responsibilities and did not make enough of the idea of shared responsibility. It was suggested that inter-vention designers had not engaged with the connections between personal responsibility and the building of safer sex as a community practice. Analysts have pointed out that the focus on individual behav-iours in much HIV prevention discourse ignores the relational context of the sexual partnership (van Campenhoudt, 1999). Research in France has attributed risky sex among gay men to individualism (Peretti-Watel et al., 2006). As I noted in Chapter 4, Flowers has suggested that HIV treatment and related technologies have led to a "fracturing" of HIV prevention into privatised concerns that reflect individualised knowledge regarding one's health status (2001: 63). In their study of engagements with HIV bio-technologies, Rosengarten and colleagues suggested that gay men with HIV had developed "... individually tailored risk minimisation strategies" (2001: 4). The practices of sero-sorting and positioning discussed in Chapter 4 are suggestive of the involvement of bio-technologies in the fragmentation of a universal understanding of HIV prevention. Researchers in the United States have argued that HIV prevention among gay men now draws on individualism (Sheon & Crosby, 2004). For example, one of their respondents is reported as having said: "... everybody takes care of themselves now" (2004: 2116). Similarly, a researcher in Australia has suggested that the notion of safer sex as collective practice and the mutual obligation it implies is no longer relevant for generations of gay men who made their sexual debut in the 1990s and 2000s (Ridge, 2004). In Canada and with reference to gay men who labelled themselves as barebackers, Adam has argued that an assumption of caveat emptor (buyer beware) informs whether or not some gay men use condoms (2005). In these situations, it is assumed that each individual has sovereignty over their own sexual health. Sexual practice that might expose them to HIV is regarded as a personal responsibility. Such negotiations are said to rely on a neo-liberal approach to civil society, which under-cuts forms of mutual obligation.

However, it may not be the case that expressions of individualism are always neo-liberal. As noted in Chapter 2, Novas and Rose found that people with Huntington's Chorea appreciated new, genetic, diagnostic tests because these allowed them to make decisions about their own life, including those that concerned their relationships with others (2000). In this view, the tests did appeal to a self-determining, some would say, entrepreneurial subject. But the tests were also valued because they allowed actors to exercise some ethical choice regarding relationships. In relation to the experience of HIV treatment, Holt and Stephenson have argued that psychological assumptions regarding the individual do further neo-liberalism (2006). According to them, the self-regulatory imperative of psychological individualism meshes with neo-liberalism and in particular the intensification of individual moral responsibility for health and wellbeing. However, as Holt and Stephenson also observe:

> ... using psy knowledge implies a degree of 'surrender' to psy terms, definitions and modes of conduct. This can render the subject more docile, more open to surveillance and regulation, but it can also

offer the subject new ways of viewing the self and different forms of conduct (2006: 214).

The individualising aspects of psychological knowledge can help create self-subjection along neo-liberal lines. However, people with HIV appear to have contested and played with psychological knowledge in a creative manner. As Holt and Stephenson suggest, there exist: "... ambiguities and inconsistencies of psychological terminology that make it a rich and productive resource for expressing the ambiguities and uncertainties of living with HIV in the contemporary period" (Holt & Stephenson, 2006: 228). This analysis suggests how forms of knowledge regarding the individual provide the basis for increased autonomy that may not necessarily, or always, extend the neo-liberal self. This perspective contrasts therefore with Adam's notion of the neo-liberal self in the discourse of gay men who have sex that might transmit HIV. Such a contrast may have to do with the focus of Holt and Stephenson on the treatment of HIV and Adam on the prevention of HIV. It may be that individualism has different expressions and uses in clinical medicine and public health governance.

As I discussed in a previous chapter, it would also be a mistake to assume that late modern forms of public health do not also retain an appeal to altruism and other imperatives that imply social obligation. For example, some commentators have argued for a focus on altruism in responses to HIV risk, such as the idea that interventions should "... promote norms of responsibility and protection of others in sexual matters" (Marks et al., 1999: 303). Such calls may reflect responses to the pernicious effects of individualism. But they may also represent attempts to accommodate people with HIV infection in public health governance. As such, they imply the reformulation of public health imperatives in relation to bio-technological knowledge, as I discussed in Chapter 5. Valentine and Waldby and colleagues have demonstrated in relation to blood donation and the risk of infectious diseases, that donors recognised the value of altruism as giving and altruism as withholding (Valentine, 2005; Waldby et al., 2004). Public health therefore is more properly considered as a flux of individualism and social obligation open to reconfiguration, partly in relation to changes in scientific knowledge and technological innovation. Elsewhere, I have questioned the idea of a straightforward individualism in HIV prevention in research with gay men HIV (Davis, 2008). In this research, the use of condoms was not managed only on the basis of individualism. As I noted in Chapter 5, HIV prevention was informed by a notion of cooperation, an approach to safer sex that resembles the relational ethics of online intimate life. HIV prevention was negotiated in the sense that it was jointly organised and resembles the safer sex as collective practice that according to some has fallen away in the face of individualism.

These questions concerning individualism connect with a more general one concerning agency and constraint in sexual citizenship. Both Plummer and Weeks have argued that the history of sexual and intimate life of the 20ᵗʰ century is one of the gradual loosening of constraints (Plummer, 2003; Weeks, 2007). But as these authors have pointed out, increased autonomy with regard to sexuality needs to be recognised as separate to individualism. Weeks in particular points out that 'cultural pessimists' of both the conservative and radical kind are joined together in their misinterpretation of this relationship. Conservatives argue that the 20ᵗʰ century has seen unprecedented loss of social obligation coupled with moral degeneracy. Radicals see in freedom new forms of coercive power pivoting around forms of rationalistic action and, in particular, neo-liberalism. Both these positions give rise to a kind of bleak picture of late modernity comprised of the deepening of negative moral judgements on difference and diversity, the furthering of false consciousness that makes individuals amenable to ideological manipulation, and the fragmentation of society into atomised social actors. In this dim light, forms of technosexuality such as internet-mediated barebacking become particularly problematic. But this negative picture does not accord with theoretical and empirical research. Referring to theorists of reflexive modernisation such as the Beck and Adkins, Weeks argued that there is a paradox in being asked to make choices about one's intimate life. The necessity of reflexive action is simultaneously constraint and opportunity. As Weeks put it: " ... choice is always limited by the social forces that have made it available" (2007: 126). This paradox is said to force a 'self-confrontation' with questions of 'How shall I be'. But such self-engagement does not mean that intimate and sexual life has been completely given over to atomised social action of the neo-liberal kind. Weeks cited research with young people in the United Kingdom which shows that they combine ideas of autonomy with notions of building relationships and therefore that the sexual self is understood as a duality of autonomy and social ties (2007: 172). Drawing on the narrative perspective, Plummer pointed out that stories of intimate life are simultaneously individual and relational (Plummer, 2003: 107–108). Reflections on the autonomous self are therefore not necessarily forms of social atomisation. Such narratives concern the positioning of the self in relation to others, which can be taken to be a practice of reflection on the ethics of intimate and sexual life.

This view regarding autonomy and constraint shifts attention away from transgression and the atomisation of sexual practice, towards a focus on the contestation of the relational ethics of sexual practice. For example, Douglas Crimp has documented a struggle in gay communities in the United States with regard to sexual responsibility and the HIV epidemic (2002). In this debate, some gay men have argued that the HIV epidemic can be attributed to the emotional immaturity and promiscuity of gay men. This line of argument accords with the more general one of the moral disarray of late modern times. Against such conservative views, Crimp has argued that gay community responses to HIV and AIDS were possible because of how such communities constituted themselves: "... AIDS didn't make gay men grow up and become responsible. AIDS showed anyone willing to pay attention how genuinely ethical the invention of gay life had been" (2002: 16). Likewise Weeks has observed how the HIV epidemic required a form of social organisation that permitted: "... the need for both individual fulfilment and for mutual involvement" (Weeks, 1998: 44). For Crimp and Weeks, safer sex is precisely a mixture of autonomy and obligation figured around the shared expectation of the avoidance of HIV transmission.

Conclusion

In this chapter, I have extended my argument for a reorientation of the typical account of internet-mediated sexual practices, and therefore technosexuality in general. Such practices are quite often regarded as problematic in so far as people hide and misrepresent themselves, and in general threaten the public good. A central concept here, and previously, has been anonymity. My argument has been that we need to let go of the idea of anonymity as a useful way of understanding internet-mediated sexual practices. Based on previous discussions of the cyber-ethnographies of intimate and sexual life, e-dating, and how such practices intersect with bio-technologies, I have argued for the idea of visibility under public health governance. By this I mean that the internet in particular is best understood as a method of making the individual visible and therefore governable. In this line of argument, anonymity is merely a form of ungovernable visibility. Some public health researchers have considered anonymity as a possible challenge for the prevention of sexually transmitted infections and HIV. However, the general shape of public health engagements with technosexuality suggests that it too is exploiting the visibility that is possible through the internet. I take the position that visibility is an epistemic strategy for public health governance. It is epistemic in the sense that it supplies a way of visualising sexual practices, or more particularly, intentions regarding sexual practices that are thought to have implications for the transmission of sexually transmitted infections and HIV. It therefore supposedly permits the monitoring of such practices and gives rise to calls for the regulation of them as matters of public policy.

I also made the point that the technosexual visibility episteme of public health governance appears to be caught up with barebacking stories. I referred to this turning as 'spectacular risk' to engage with its visibility, its transgressive extremity, and the way in which such a form of risk-taking operates as the source of its own proof. Like others, I have suggested that barebacking is a moral panic and that some public health researchers have so far failed to recognise it as such. Spectacular risk also shows how the bio-technological mediation of sexual practices is being debated. It suggests how technosexual visibility can be exploited as a kind of pornography of transgression, which can reinforce the position of technosexuality as outside acceptable boundaries of sexual practice. It thus lends itself to a forensic orientation in research and intervention. However, if we can accept the idea that technosexual visibility is amenable to public health governance, it is also possible to consider this relationship in reverse. In the next chapter therefore, I want to explore the idea that technosexuality may be changing public health.

7
The Reshaping of Public Health

The previous chapter explored the idea that public health governance can exploit technosexual visibility. In Chapter 5, I explored how public health governance tries to exert itself through various imperatives and how these articulate with bio-technologies. These chapters have therefore addressed public health governance and how it impinges on, or works through, technosexuality. In this chapter, I want to consider how technosexuality may help to (re)shape public health governance. Superficially, it would be possible to argue that the ways in which some forms of public health governance seek to exploit technosexuality is a simple process of medicalisation, or in other terms, the incorporation of technosexual citizens into a form of total society public health governance, extended to bio- and communication technologies and their hybrids. But it may be a simplification to conclude that public health only extends its authority through technosexual practices. Drawing on the example of the Viagra cyborg and the productively disruptive effects it is said to have in relation to medical authority and sexual embodiment, this chapter considers how technosexuality may be altering the social relations of public health governance. As we will see, the decentring implied in these changes raises the prospect of a paradoxical extension and loosening of public health authority over technosexuality.

As I suggested in Chapter 2, Viagra scholarship has argued for a complex medicalisation and de-medicalisation of sexual embodiment and relations. The rise of the Viagra user is said to reflect a relay of social relations with regard to bio-technology that exhibits a strengthened relationship between bio-technology consumers and providers, and therefore a decentring of the power of medical authority. This arrangement of consumer, prescriber, provider suggests a reduction in medicalisation of, for example, sexuality, and therefore the expansion of democratic possibilities for the intersection of sexual practice, technology and public health governance. Alternatively, this arrangement of consumer, prescriber, provider may lead to novel forms of re-medicalisation that may not in the end have much benefit for consumers as such, and perhaps mask the operation of forms of exploitation. As I have noted, HIV treatment advocacy has been considered as an example of techno-democracy. Although some provisions apply, it has been argued that HIV treatment advocacy has addressed medical power, by questioning the accepted forms of clinical practice and treatments research (Epstein, 2000). But it also seems to be the case that treatment advocacy can lead to forms of re-medicalisation, as advocates become incorporated into forms of authority.

Medicalisation has long been understood to imply the countervailing process of de-medicalisation. Medicalisation can be defined as the process where practices and identities are defined in medical terms, therefore placing them under the control of medical authority. In crude terms, de-medicalisation can be understood as the weakening of an explicitly medical authority over health. Ivan Illich noted how both medicalisation and de-medicalisation were necessary responses to the burgeoning complexity and costs of health care in the late modern period (1975). Illich argued that modern systems of health care extend medical power by disseminating diagnostic and treatment techniques throughout society. Naming new domains of social action as medical problems enlarge forms of medical authority. Public health governance accords with this pattern by defining technosexuality as a problem but also exploiting it as a means of governance. However, the expansion of the definitions of what counts as disease, and in particular, the incorporation of more social actors into the systems of power that grant the authority over such definitions, inevitably leads to a diffusion and fragmentation of authority to call such disease categories into being and govern through them. For example, health promotion seeks to educate the population with regard to such concerns as diet and exercise, by circulating knowledge and expertise and co-opting institutions into interventions. In such strategies, school teachers and parents may be asked to take on the role of addressing childhood obesity. The inclusion of teachers and parents in the promotion of healthy diets and exercise means that they may gain authority to speak and act for the governance of health. Teachers and parents therefore become sources of authority in public health. In this way, medicalisation inevitably provides the seeds for de-medicalisation, or at least, the basis for contesting absolute, institutional, medical authority. Debate hinges on whether such processes redistribute authority in ways that promote democratic forms of health governance, or simply spread medical power in the guise of other forms of knowledge and institutional arrangements.

In this chapter therefore, I want to consider medicalisation and the related process of de-medicalisation, to assess the scope for democratic expressions of the public health governance of technosexuality. In the following sections, I discuss the theoretical background of medicalisation in more detail, with particular reference to the rise of the health product consumer. I then discuss medicalisation and related concepts, assessing how these concepts can be made relevant for the case of technosexuality and public health governance. Based on this consideration of technosexuality and public health authority, in the last section of this chapter I reflect on the democratic possibilities of a technologically-mediated public health governance. As I will argue, a simple notion of democracy has limitations, but a dialogical form of public health may have merit.

Authority and public health

As Illich and many others have pointed out, medicalisation is not a one-way process of encroachment on social practices and the subordination of individuals and institutions. De-medicalisation is also implied in the spreading network of medicalised knowledge, practices and institutions. It is likely that public health follows this pattern. Further, the bio- and communication technologies that are important to technosexuality may help extend both medicalisation and de-medicalisation. Throughout this book, I have emphasised that both bio- and communication technologies are relevant to sexually transmitted infections and HIV. I have also argued that bio- and communication technologies are expressed in hybrid forms in technosexuality. Likewise, it is important to recognise how communication technologies are extended by bio-technologies and vice versa. The internet finds extra value in its capacity to make bio-technological knowledge and products available. Bio-technologisation is in part achieved through its alignment with communication technologies that are used to understand and access it, and as I have shown, extend its effects into social and sexual life. As this book has aimed to establish, there are many ways in which public health is exploiting such technologies and their hybrids. To take one particularly mediatised example, researchers have reported on the findings of an online survey of gay men, evaluating the health benefits of a story-line regarding syphilis in the popular medical soap 'ER' (Whittier et al., 2005). This example supports Plummer's point that our life experience is saturated with mediatised sexual narratives (2003). In this case however, we could say that the life experience of citizens is also becoming saturated with public health narratives. We can recognise in this example, that public health governance is not restricted to institutions named as such. The media are also involved, suggesting that they have a role to play in medicalisation and de-medicalisation. These perspectives underline the notion of public health as total society governance (Petersen & Lupton, 1996). In this section therefore, I want to consider two perspectives that help shed light on how networks of multiple actors have become implicated in processes of medicalisation and de-medicalisation. One is the Foucauldian inspired notion of surveillance medicine said to involve the reconfiguration of medical power by disseminating its techniques, knowledge, and effects throughout the social body (Armstrong, 1995). Risk, discussed in Chapter 5 in connection with public health imperatives, provides another way of conceptualising such changes. Although it is important to recognise that it is not regarded as compatible with surveillance medicine, risk does provide a contrast with the Foucauldian school by drawing attention to different concerns, in particular, trust and security (Lupton, 1999). In different ways, these two perspectives suggest that, partly through bio- and communication technology, medicine has become disseminated as a condition of all our lives, with consequent changes in the status of medical authority as the only and trusted source of such knowledge and expertise. I also want to introduce Mary-Jo Delvecchio-Good's notion of the 'bio-technical embrace', because it helps develop the notion of medicalisation/de-medicalisation in relation to bio-technological innovation.

Surveillance medicine is based on the idea that changes in the conceptualisation of health and illness have altered how medicine is practised. Briefly, scholars have argued that the medical focus on the sick body has been replaced by the notion of pre-disposing or lifestyle factors (Armstrong, 1993). Surveillance medicine has been referred to as a "... network of visibility" (Armstrong, 1995: 395), echoing the visibility of technosexuals under public health governance. Accumulating information concerning the distribution of disease in populations, technological developments, and shifts in how societies are governed in general, have created the conditions for a form of medicine that exists outside the clinic and the hospital. Individuals have increasingly been asked to regulate their own health by making adjustments in their environments, daily habits, health care regimens, parenting practices and so on. Surveillance medicine therefore works to produce a " ... health promoting self" (Nettle-ton & Bunton, 1995: 50). Part of this rationality involves the internal-isation of the method of surveillance of populations. Individuals take on self-surveillance, establishing themselves as vigilant subjects and there-fore also placing themselves into systems of surveillance medicine. The boundary of the hospital as the focus of health care has dissolved, or at least become much more permeable, to make way for preventative forms of medicine. Increasingly, ex-clinic medical services have been located in places such as schools and the workplace and, via the shaping of the prac-tices of individuals themselves, into the quotidian realm itself. Internet-mediated forms of health care and public health intervention can be taken as examples of the dissemination of medical self-surveillance. The focus in this form of medicine becomes the 'expert' patient. This is a notional patient understood as knowledgeable, rational and capable of mastering themselves and their health and wellbeing. Public health gov-ernance is in some respects the idealised expression of surveillance medi-cine. As Petersen has pointed out, the notion of the expert patient is important in public health because it performs the function of joining the individual to the state (1996). In this view, the putative self-governing patient is nevertheless tied to forms of direct governance through their reliance on systems of authority and expert knowledge managed and dis-seminated by state-run institutions. But as I have demonstrated, other institutions, such as the media and commercial organisations, are also invested in public health governance.

In Chapter 5, I discussed risk as one major public health imperative. Compared with surveillance medicine, risk has a different way of concep-tualising health subjectivity. Like surveillance medicine, risk society also addresses the knowledgeable, self-regulating patient, but in a way that emphasises the challenges of trust and security for a relatively auto-nomous social actor, as opposed to self-subjection under health gover-nance. For example, each of us has to make prudent decisions about our relationships, parenting and working life. But such decisions are rarely simply 'yes or no'. We are often called upon to make choices when we are uncertain of outcomes. In addition, other kinds of uncertainties are rife in late modernity. Scientific knowledge and the effects of technology are never 'black and white'. For example, medical interventions are often couched in terms of risks. If you have ever had major surgery or embarked on treatment, your doctor may have discussed benefits and dangers. Uncertainties such as these can affect life decisions and have implications for emotional wellbeing. As I have shown in the preceding chapters, public health efforts concerning sexually transmitted infections and HIV are often couched in terms of risk calculations and therefore a general appeal to a rational and risk averse social actor.

The notions of surveillance medicine and risk society furnish perspectives regarding the reorganisation of the social relations of health care in late modern times. However, these perspectives, as I have described them, do not explain why these changes have occurred. These perspectives are missing the element of subjectivity that can explain why all these social actors are joined in the name of health in general or health technology in particular. To find a contender for this missing element, we can to turn to Delvecchio-Good's notion of the 'bio-technical embrace' (2001). Based on interviews with cancer patients, observations of clinical encounters, and analysing the products of a cyberspace network of bone marrow transplant patients (BMT-talk), Delvecchio-Good has conceptualised the bio-technical embrace as so:

> ... the metaphoric language of many patients is profoundly affective, expressing hope and interest in the possibilities of biotechnical innovations and therapeutics, whether in consultation with their clinicians discussing therapeutic choices, results, and ambiguities or in the less structured interviews with researchers. In BMT-talk, cyberspace connections often appear to heighten the emotionality of discourses and graphic debates with patients over limits to therapeutic options. The affective dimensions of high-technology medicine are clearly soteriological, a salvation ethos that is fundamental to bioscience and biomedicine, and to the political economy and culture of hope. The biotechnical embrace creates a popular culture enamored with the biology of hope, attracting venture capital that continues even in the face of contemporary constraints to generate new treatment modalities (2001: 407).

The bio-technical embrace is the meta-narrative of TV medical soaps, health news reporting, the accounts of clinicians, and stories of lived experience. Significantly, Delvecchio-Good has made the point that commercial organisations involved in bio-technologies draw on this narrative to secure their position in the bio-technology economy. Patients, clinicians and commercial organisations are therefore joined together under the meta-narrative of the bio-technical embrace.

Medicalisation and de-medicalisation

A superficial reading of the notion of the self-regulating patient conceptualised through these concepts of surveillance medicine or risk society, would be that bio- and communication technology provide the means by which public health can extend its authority over individuals, or in other words, medicalise technosexuality. For example, surveillance medicine implies that the individual is required to subject themselves to medical discourse. From the risk society point of view, the proliferation of scientific and clinical knowledge derived from biotechnology, leads to uncertainty for the patient, producing a kind of iatrogenic medicalisation. The biology of hope narrative gives such forms of medicalisation their ideational force. But as I have already suggested, there is cause to argue that de-medicalisation is also possible. Further, in some circumstances, forms of medical authority can aid in the pursuit of social justice. It also seems possible to argue that technosexuality has a special role to play in these processes of medicalisation and de-medicalisation.

Bio-technologies that have implications for sexual practice can lend themselves to a specific intensification of medicalisation and de-medicalisation. Critical studies of Viagra, Cialis and Levitra have taken these pharmaceutical products to be examples of medicalisation (Bass, 2001; Conrad & Leiter, 2004; Marshall, 2007; Wienke, 2006). As I discussed in Chapter 2, the core of this medicalisation argument is that, before Viagra, erectile dysfunction was regarded as a psychological problem. But after Viagra, erectile dysfunction is understood as a biological problem that can be addressed by bio-technology. In this way an aspect of sexual experience is redefined in bio-technological terms, incorporating sexual experience into systems of medical authority and control. The effort to find a treatment for female sexual dysfunction can be taken as another example of medicalisation (Hartley, 2006). But as I also discussed in Chapter 2, the exercise of the Viagra cyborg is in fact not always in the hands of clinicians. To some extent, Viagra displaces medical authority because, due to the manner in which erections and orgasms generally escape the medical gaze, it is a self-prescribed technology, both in the clinic and through the internet. In this sense, Viagra is the ideal pharmaceutical product for the production of patient consumers, because the power of medical authority over the body of the patient is suspended, or at least, somewhat deflected. In this regard, Viagra could be said to be an example of de-medicalisation. It can also be argued that surveillance medicine and heightened awareness of risk have themselves contributed to the diminution or at least reconfiguration of medical authority. The idea that individuals are now asked to take on their own health care, radically alters how medical authority is understood and exercised. The iatrogenic effects of bio-technologies raise anxieties concerning the negative aspects of medical care. The emergence of multi-drug resistant infections, such as in the case HIV (Salomon et al., 2000), have created problems for patients and prescribers and the extension of the medical domination of body and society.

It is therefore not strictly tenable to rely on a medicalisation thesis as a way of understanding the relationship between technosexuality and public health governance. It seems more likely that a useful conceptual framework is de-medicalisation coupled with bio-technologisation (Rosenfeld & Faircloth, 2006; Webster, 2007). As Rosenfeld and Faircloth and Webster have pointed out, de-medicalisation combined with bio-technologisation implies that medical authority has become decentred as the main or only source of authority over the body and health, but at the same time, bio-technologies and the knowledge that is required to use them are no less important, or even more important, in the daily lives of individuals. On this basis we can make a distinction between de-medicalisation and bio-technologisation (Webster, 2007). De-medicalisation refers to the processes where medical authority is questioned, decentred or displaced by other systems of authority such as patient power and commercial organisations. Bio-technologisation concerns the redefinition of life and social relations through biological and technological innovation. It also needs to be recognised that bio-technologies are not restricted to the institutional context of medicine. While they can mediate medical authority of health and the body, they mediate other forms of power, such as that of commercial organisations or consumers themselves.

It is also possible to argue that Viagra and related products break down a medical model of sexual embodiment and suggest democratic engagements with bio-technologies. For example, users of Viagra do not necessarily adopt a biomedical model of erectile dysfunction, but they nevertheless appreciate the effects of the technology itself (Potts et al., 2006). Viagra can also be understood as a form of bio-technologisation that has reduced the stigma of erectile dysfunction by making it acceptable to use treatment, and therefore extracted the dysfunctional sexual body from medical authority (Potts et al., 2004). To take an example from another area, some have argued that the internet is transforming the science, marketing and prescribing of psychoactive medications (Cohen et al., 2001). Because the internet permits interactivity, it helps the patient gain knowledge regarding their mental health drugs that would ordinarily have been restricted to professionals. The internet is therefore said to foster a participatory medicine where patients become actors in the "... construction of knowledge about medications" (Cohen et al., 2001: 454).

But others have cautioned that we should not oversimplify the notion of de-medicalisation or under-estimate the value of traditional forms of medical authority (Ettorre et al., 2006). Purdy charted a feminist interpretation of processes of de-medicalisation with reference to institutional practice rather than knowledge (2001). Purdy suggested that medical definitions of health and embodiment remain useful because at times they are needed as the basis for access to goods and services, particularly in health economies that rely on private health insurance. Purdy therefore made a distinction between the problem of the cultural arrangement of medical practices that further paternalism and other forms of coercive power, and the democratisation of useful biomedical knowledge, expertise and effects. In research regarding medicalisation and pharmaceutical products including Viagra, Conrad and Leiter have argued that while the centre of power has shifted, medicine remains a dominant force (2004). Conrad and Leiter note that the medicalisation of erectile dysfunction predates Viagra, so it is a mistake to assume that Viagra is singly the technology that has medicalised the male sexual body.

There is also critical inquiry in the area of sexual citizenship that has retrieved medical authority for the purposes of social justice. Matthew Waites has considered how medicalised notions of the cause of homosexuality remain important in politics and law (2005). Waites has recognised that medical knowledge regarding the causes of homosexuality is not internally stable and has been hotly contested in terms of unwanted effects in the lives of lesbians and gay men, among others. Nevertheless notions of the medical and biological causes of sexual difference have, from time to time, been useful in the political fight for the sexual autonomy. Waites pointed out that, because such explanations naturalise sexual difference, homosexuality achieves a kind of re-medicalisation that works to provide the basis for assured citizenship status. Therefore it would be a mistake to argue that the medicalisation of sexual difference is problematic in an absolute sense. Waites therefore provides a picture of a more strategic and dialogical employment of medical and biological concepts regarding sexual desire, and a kind of appropriation of medicine and bio-technology as a matter of sexual autonomy and social justice. This dialogical pattern can be taken to characterise the history of medicine and sexuality, as medical authority over sexuality has at times been useful for, and at times destructive of, sexual autonomy. In this regard, Waites sits at odds with Halperin discussed in Chapter 1, who does seem to want to argue for the unnecessary medicalisation, or specifically psycho-pathologisation, of gay men's sexuality. In light of Waites's analysis, perhaps we could say that Halperin's argument is one moment in this dialogue concerning medical knowledge and sexuality.

It may also be that forms of technosexuality have been central to these complex processes of medicalisation, de-medicalisation, and bio-technologisation. For example, the contraceptive Pill has been discussed in terms of medicalisation, but also in a way that suggests it is involved in de-medicalisation and bio-technologisation. Hera Cook has argued that the Pill enhanced the autonomy of women in sexual relations, fertility and participation in the labour market, but that it also led to some challenges for women (2005). For example, because the Pill allowed women to delay pregnancy, women could stay longer in the work-place. However, the knowledge that the Pill prevented pregnancy led some men to expect that women were available for sexual intercourse (Cook, 2005: 121). Importantly for this present argument, the introduction of the Pill demonstrates changes in medical control over sexuality and the reconfiguration of sexuality and technology. As Cook revealed, the Pill was unlike previous forms of contraceptive technology, such as condoms and diaphragms, because it required a prescription and therefore a consultation with a medical practitioner. The introduction of the Pill therefore forced a relationship between medical authority and the sexual practice of heterosexual couples, seemingly reinforcing the medicalisation of sexuality. However, Cook revealed a countervailing account where medical paternalism and moral restraint ironically laid the groundwork for a very different arrangement of sexual action, bio-technology and medical authority. Medical practitioners in the United Kingdom were at first reluctant to prescribe the Pill as part of the National Health Service on the grounds that scant state resources should not be used for facilitating the sexual pleasure of the heterosexual couple. This moral position seems reminiscent of the one that informed approaches to syphilis, as I discussed in Chapter 5. This reluctance meant that for a time women had to fund their own prescriptions for the Pill. It seems that sexuality, and specifically sexual pleasure, was placed outside of the central activity of medical care, and was therefore positioned as a domain of self-determination. According to Cook, medical practitioners were also able to negotiate an increase in fees for the onerous duty of prescribing the Pill, a kind of bounty for servicing the now burgeoning growth in demand for a bio-technology that was seen to promote sexual pleasure. Women themselves actively challenged medical expertise, for example, when doctors dismissed the side effects of oral contraceptives as psychogenic. Cook's account therefore gives the impression of the gradual reconfiguration of medical authority over the sexual bodies of women, but without a lessening of the importance of the technology itself and biological understandings of the body and health care. This double manoeuvre in relation to the Pill supports notions of de-medicalisation. Strikingly, it also rather strongly suggests that questions of sexuality have taken a central position in such processes. The view that sexual pleasure is private, or even vice, and therefore a domain for self-determination, is one of the assumptions that furthers de-medicalisation. In this view therefore, technosexuality is not a side-show in medicalisation and de-medicalisation. Instead, we need to consider the idea that forms of technosexuality are in fact pivotal to such processes because of the specific manner in which they join up, and invite the re-configuration of: the dominion of the sovereign, pleasuring self; medical authority; and technological innovation.

Democratic health care?

The decentring of medical authority and rise of the knowledgeable, self-regulating patient, particularly in relation to technosexuality, suggests that more egalitarian practices of health care are possible. But, as others have argued in relation to health care in general, it also seems that the knowledgeable, self-regulating patient provides a method for extending medical authority in novel ways that are not necessarily commensurate with democracy. In particular, it seems that the notional self-regulating patient functions as a bridgehead for medical authority in a bio-technologically mediated health care system, and also provides the basis for the insertion of commercial interests. These perspectives imply that the public health governance of technosexuality is also subject to hidden forms of power and, perhaps, exploitation.

Several researchers have taken up the question of whether the internet can provide the basis for the democratisation of health care. For example, Hardey has interviewed householders in the United Kingdom concerning how they used the internet to manage everyday health concerns (1999). Hardey argued that the self-directed, discerning use of online medical information was empowering for lay users. On that basis he suggested that lay access to such information contributed to de-medicalisation and therefore that an egalitarian form of health care was coming into being through the internet.

However, not all researchers have reached the conclusion that the internet promotes health democracy. Also addressing the challenges for the individual in ehealth, Cullen and Cohn have discussed internet-mediated health services in the United Kingdom (2006). Cullen and Cohn pointed out the great complexity of the online health services that have recently been introduced. For example, there is a proliferation of: government supported services; general health information sites; specialised sites established by communities of interest, such as in the areas of sexual health and HIV; specialised sites established by public health institutions, charities, and corporations. Such complexity reveals multiple players and the interplay of government, commerce and affected communities. Cullen and Cohn referred to HIV as an example of how individuals affected by a health issue have influenced the production of knowledge and services, and therefore become players in ehealth. As I noted in Chapter 4, the HIV treatment advocacy movement has been regarded as an important force in changing the practice of clinical research regarding HIV bio-technologies. The advocacy movement is now occupied with ensuring that people with HIV have up-to-date information regarding HIV bio-technologies (see for example: *aidsmap.com* and *thebody.com*). Cullen and Cohn conceptualised these public health systems as socially embedded techno-action systems where lay people and experts work together. As Cullen and Cohn suggest, such systems have benefits in terms of: increased access to information; overcoming social isolation, especially for people with rare or stigmaed health issues such as sexually transmitted infections and HIV; access to peer advice and emotional support; skilling up patients in readiness for clinical encounters; giving professionals insight into the life world of patients; promoting the value of psychosocial care in relation to public health concerns. But Cullen and Cohn also argued that ehealth is not necessarily democratising. Their content analysis of online discussions in women's health forums revealed that particular 'individuals' appeared to be in fact promoting products to other discussants, and may have been employed by companies promoting health products. So while the internet gives patients and carers access to information and support it also opens them up to the interests of commercial organisations. In an analysis of the marketing of a treatment for HIV infection in the United Kingdom, where direct to consumer marketing is not permitted, Rosengarten has shown that pharmaceutical companies rely on various methods of influencing patients, including: treatment information magazines written by and for people with HIV, mainstream news stories, and advertising in medical journals to prescribers (2004). Rosengarten made the point that, because these sources of knowledge are trusted, this kind of promotion strategy can be more influential than direct marketing.

As noted in Chapter 2, Fox and Ward have taken up a critique of the notion of the knowledgeable, self-regulating patient in relation to what they describe as the: "... increasingly industrialised, technology-driven, consumer oriented and media saturated global health and illness economy" (Fox & Ward, 2006: 477). Their work was based on case studies of ehealth, including Viagra. They used a Deleuzian framework of becoming embodiment, which gives rise to the notion of "healthing-bodies" as they put it (Fox & Ward, 2006: 475). By this they mean that: "... health identities are neither prior, nor are they determined. Rather they emerge from concrete embodiment practices in relation to material, cultural, technological and emotional contexts" (Fox & Ward, 2006: 475). For Fox and Ward, the idea of the relatively autonomous patient is fictive and operates as a method for ensuring the extension of medical authority by furthering responsible compliance on the part of patients. The notion of the knowledgeable, self-regulating patient therefore provides a way of masking and extending the importance of medical authority over health, even through the putative, self-determining practices of people using the internet.

Nettleton and Hanlon have also argued against the self-determining patient in research regarding ehealth behaviour and use of NHS Direct in the United Kingdom (Nettleton & Hanlon, 2006). In line with Fox and Ward, they argued that the patient conceived of as knowledgeable and free is in effect a form of compliance with medical authority. NHS Direct is a United Kingdom internet and call centre technology that provides the general public access to clinical advice regarding common health problems. NHS Direct is designed to help lay people seek simple treatment and, if need be, medical consultation. It is also based on the assumption of the knowledgeable, self-regulating patient, seeking and using advice provided by health professionals. Nettleton and Hanlon argued that the social process of accessing medical expertise is not wholly altered by information technologies, although some reconfiguration is possible. For example, interviewees reported that they used NHS Direct to make decisions about whether or not they should take the step of visiting a clinician because they did not want to waste the time of busy professionals. In this regard, the online health care services worked to protect traditional institutional arrangements that support medical authority, and not necessarily to create egalitarian health care. Likewise, in qualitative interviews with women regarding how they engaged with knowledge regarding hormone replacement treatment, Henwood and colleagues argued that the notion of a knowledgeable, self-regulating patient masks the true operation of power

(2003). For example, not all women actively sought out knowledge via the internet and other sources. Some preferred to rely instead on their medical practitioners. In addition, the internet itself was one among many sources of information that the women found useful. Internet-users were aware that the internet could be a misleading source of information. Some interviewees also found they were dismissed by their medical practitioners if they raised questions derived from their internet searches. Interviewees said they resolved this issue by keeping such knowledge to themselves. Henwood and colleagues argued there-fore that the idea of the democratisation of health care through the internet is utopian. In this regard, they suggest that the literacy of the patient and medical authority circumscribed ehealth democracy. They made the point that the assumption of a knowledgeable, self-determining patient of bio-technologically mediated forms of health care helps elabor-ate and extend forms of compliance with medical authority and has the effect of drawing attention away from continuing paternalism in the medical encounter.

Dialogical public health

As the previous discussion has indicated, it is not strictly possible to argue that health care is a simple form of medicalisation. Techno-sexuality itself provides examples of why this may not be the case. However, it also seems to be the case that de-medicalisation may not lead to democratic forms of health care. For example, while super-ficially attractive as a form of democracy, the idea of 'expert' patients may be a way of extending forms of medical authority in novel ways. It is also important to point out that technosexuality itself may not be democratic. As I have noted in Chapter 3, the narcissistic aspects of e-dating may inhibit the construction of democratic social relations. Gosine's analysis of racism and online communication in gay men's e-dating websites, provided an example of how e-dating can extend forms of social exclusion (2007). In addition, there is an argument that, because e-dating in general is so attached to forms of informational capitalism, its democratic virtues are questionable (Arvidsson, 2006; Smaill, 2004). These doubts are amplified if we take the view that forms of technosexuality, such as e-dating, are not just colonised by com-mercial interests, but provide a generic template for the operation of informational capitalism. The public health governance of techno-sexuality exhibits similar ambiguity. It attempts to extend its authority over and through technosexuality. But through appeals to autonomous subjects, and its network of multiple actors, public health decentres itself. We are therefore led to consider whether it is possible to entertain democratic forms of public health governance of technosexuality, or if this situation simply extends public health governance in new ways. However, as I have argued, technosexuality itself is derived from a relational ethics of reciprocal relations. It follows that there may also be scope for a relational engagement with authority pertaining to technosexuality and public health, or dialogue, as it has been sometimes called in the literature.

I have provided examples of how public health is attempting to extend authority over technosexuality. For example, it has been reported that public health practitioners in the United States have used e-dating emails to notify individuals that they may have been exposed to syphilis (Adams, 2004). This approach is justified on the basis that the apparent anonymity of e-dating does not permit traditional forms of contact tracing. Gay men's e-dating websites are now populated with pop-ups and banners advertising health education information and services. Health educators hang in chat-rooms and provide information and referral on request. Websites provide email consultations for young people seeking information and advice in relation to sexual health (Harvey et al., 2007). Some interventions for gay men are explicitly directed at encouraging: testing for sexually transmitted infections and HIV; partner notification; and behaviour change to prevent further infections (Rietmeijer & Shamos, 2007). A content analysis of existing sexual health websites in general found that the universal underlying approach was the dissemination of information and persuasion, with a focus on abstinence from sexual intercourse and condom use (Noar et al., 2006). Such strategies recognise the existence of technosexual actors, but they also exhibit a focus on using the internet to extend clinical services and sexual health education. Such interventions, in effect, concern the re-orientation of clinical and educational services and procedures directed at compliant populations. In this way an assumption is made that patients will engage with such interventions, either as passive recipients or as prudent actors.

However, there also seems to be a case for the existence of dialogical forms of engagement with public health authority regarding sexual health concerns. For example, research regarding subjectivity and HIV treatment has come to support this dialogical view. As I noted in Chapter 4, the complexities of HIV treatment have become a central challenge for people with HIV, in terms of: the risk of HIV transmission; fears regarding the ongoing effectiveness of HIV treatment technologies; and the psychosocial burden of sustaining complex and demanding treatment on a life-long basis (Green & Smith, 2004). This situation has created a focus on how people with HIV digest and apply knowledge concerning treatment technologies in terms of sexual health and health in general. A research literature in the area of HIV is focused on the correct and regular use of HIV treatment. This work hinges on the concept of treatment prescription 'adherence' (Green & Smith, 2004). This research typically documents the social and psychological co-factors of failing to comply with treatment prescriptions. In medical sociology, there is some controversy concerning the democratic possibilities of the relationships between treatment users and prescribers. For example, and echoing the e-health research already discussed, the concept of power sharing in treatment partnerships has been critiqued as masking hidden forms of power (Stevenson & Scambler, 2005). The disciplinary term 'adherence' common in the area of HIV is testimony to the high stakes of treatment failure, but also to the underlying relations of patient and medical authority in operation. We need to also recognise that there has been a historic shift from treatment advocacy to treatment adherence in the area of HIV. As I outlined in Chapter 3, it has been argued that before more effective treatment was available, medical expertise was in crisis concerning its ability to treat people with HIV, opening up a politics of treatment advocacy and encouraging experimental forms of treatment (Epstein, 1996). With the advent of effective treatment, there has been a shift to adherence. But the shift raises questions over the relationship that people with HIV have with the systems of expert knowledge that support treatment.

Sitting in contrast with the notion of treatment adherence is close focus qualitative research in the area of HIV which reveals that engagements with expertise can be relational and dialogical. Researchers in Australia have argued that patient/doctor relations are "collaborative" (Persson et al., 2003: 411). In this research, a bio-technological model of health and embodiment, particularly with regard to sexual health implications, was resisted, but also exploited in ways that permitted productive and enabling engagements with living with HIV infection. Interviews with gay men with HIV in the United Kingdom suggested that engagements with the knowledge generated by HIV bio-technologies were necessarily achieved and sustained through a relationship between the medical expert and the treatment user (Davis, 2007). As I noted in Chapter 4, HIV bio-technologies have contentious links with the risk of HIV transmission in sexual practice, for example, the idea that HIV treatment may reduce the chance of HIV transmission in sexual practice. Gay men with HIV are expected to be knowledgeable of the provisions that apply to these effects. But interviewees suggested that such knowledge could be interpreted in different ways and that the views of medical experts differed between individuals, agencies and over time. Such knowledge was therefore seen to be provisional. Gay men with HIV were also aware that misinterpreting such information could have implications for HIV transmission to their sexual partners and therefore be profoundly significant for the politics of risk and blame. Bio-technology users were found to draw medical experts into their accounts of engagements with such knowledge as a matter of dialogue between patient and doctor. Medical authority therefore had value as a source of expertise in conditions where knowledge was contentious and could change. Medical experts also had value because they were not directly implicated in the risk and blame concerning HIV transmission in sexual practice.

There are also examples of technosexuality and public health that exhibit a dialogical character. Emails sent to sexual health services by young people in the United Kingdom were analysed to explore communication with online sexual health advisors (Harvey et al., 2007). This research was used to draw attention to the employment by young people of an electronic, textual, 'genre' of sexual health communication shaped around a normative understanding of sexuality. Young people couched their communication in terms of how their sexual experiences might differ from some notion of normality. The users of the website were therefore seen to be medicalising themselves. The researchers advocated that future online consultations with such young people ought to work to moderate these forms of medicalising self-subjection, by challenging normative notions of sexuality. These researchers therefore argued that sexual health professionals should attend to this genre of normalisation in their online conversations with young people to ensure improvements in online sexual health care. It is also likely that much can be learned from understanding how people exploit forms of technosexuality themselves. Analysis of the web-pages made by Black American young women revealed the circulation of self-representations that reinforce and resist sexual stereotypes (Stokes, 2007). In particular, website-makers revealed themselves through the discourse of the 'hypersexual black person', a form of sexuality that reinforced the role of women as the objects of heterosexual men's desires. However, some of the young women chose forms of sexuality that placed expectations on male partners. These presentations of self were taken to reveal an active agency on the part of the young women and the related capacity to reflect on the racing of sexuality, gender and power. These authors made a call for increased efforts concerning critical media literacy for young people.

Further support for this dialogical viewpoint arises from the practical aspects of making online life work, as I discussed in Chapter 3. E-daters are aware of the stigma attached to online sexual practices and the possibility of sexual exploitation that exists online, as in other settings. In e-dating environments, e-daters adopted strategies of checking and verifying the images and texts of prospective dates. These strategies could extend to combining e-dating communication with other forms of interaction such a emailing, messaging, SMS texting, and even telephone calls. I noted how some e-daters can exploit the forms of communication made available in e-dating websites to pre-empt social rejection. Like questing avatars, e-daters experimented with self-presentation as a method for testing out their prospective dates. E-daters therefore appear to have a repertoire of techno-social skills that involve the articulation of informational and symbolic resources.

However, we are only beginning to understand this hermeneutics of technosexual existence. Research has shown that gay men with HIV can pre-empt the stigma attached to HIV positive serostatus by making their own status explicit or implied in online communication (Davis et al., 2006c). In addition, such men seemed aware of the turning in risk culture that assigns blame to people with HIV. For that reason, disclosing HIV serostatus could be taken to work to moderate such blame. Gay men in general can also make their HIV prevention intentions explicit in online communication. For example, some websites allow users to code their preference for use of condoms by operating radio buttons to indicate: 'never'; 'sometimes'; 'always'; 'needs discussion'. In some circumstances, online communication was used to establish serosameness, therefore giving rise to forms of sexual interaction that moderated questions of stigma, blame and HIV transmission. But as Race has pointed out, such negotiations are 'fragile' and depend on the critical literacy of its participants (2003). In online research of homosexually-interested, heterosexual men, Pryce has made reference to the "... pedagogy of the cybersexual" (2008: 137) to point out that so far we know little about the eliteracy that actors bring to technosexuality or how the skills are acquired that make such online life possible. Cyberethnographies and critical studies of technosexuality have so far only summarised the general pattern of, for example the relational ethics of questing avatars, or the existence of Viagra cyborgs and the related implications for sexual embodiment and systems of medical authority. If there is merit in addressing the public health governance of technosexuality through dialogical forms of authority, it is necessary to engage with the related concerns of literacy and pedagogy.

Conclusion

This chapter has explored the wider implications of technosexuality and public health governance with reference to theoretical debates regarding medical authority in bio-technologically mediated forms of health care. I took this route of inquiry because I wanted to consider the (re)configuration of power in the public health governance of technosexuality. This chapter therefore complements the previous two, which have explored public health imperatives applied to technosexuality, and the exercise of public health through the visibility of technosexuality. With reference to concepts from surveillance medicine, risk, and Delvecchio-Good's notion of the bio-technical embrace, I have suggested how the processes of medicalisation and de-medicalisation implicate multiple actors in public health governance joined under the promise of technological innovation. These actors include, patient/consumers, medical practitioners, public health practitioners, public institutions charged with sexual health care, and possibly even commercial organisations invested in forms of technosexuality. Power in relation to public health governance of technosexuality is understood as a relay of relationships between these actors. Partly because of the ways in which it is seeking to address technosexuality, public health can be thought of as constituted in the relays and networks of multiple actors, including, patients, clinicians, government, media and commercial organisations. In a sense then, there is no 'public' outside these social relations.

It is possible to argue that technosexuality is the means by which such complexities of de-medicalisation come into being. Forms of technosexuality supply the logic, or at least a particularly intense instance, of de-medicalisation. Technosexual forms, such as Viagra and the contraceptive Pill, create connections between the idea of sexual pleasure as a domain for individual volition, the suspension of medical authority over such aspects of sexuality, technological innovation, and commercial activity. In addition, re-medicalisation also appeared to have value, because in some circumstances it permitted the pursuit of social justice for sexual citizens. I have considered critical perspectives regarding the notional knowledgeable, self-regulating patient and how, in general, this identity extends the exercise of medical power but not always in ways that were antithetical to patient wellbeing. With reference to e-health in general, I noted that the notional autonomous patient, understood as in a relay with systems of medical authority, appears to be a kind of bridgehead for forms of re-medicalisation. I argued, however, that technosexual actors could take up dialogues with systems of biotechnological knowledge where the ongoing management of relationships with representatives of medical authority becomes important.

Previous chapters have demonstrated how public health governance addresses and exercises itself through technosexuality. This chapter has argued that some features of technosexuality may be driving the reconfiguration of public health governance and modifying its authority over the management of sexually transmitted infections. I also suggested that there may be scope for dialogical engagements with such systems of public health authority. A dialogical form of public health in technosexuality may not be dominant. Indeed, some public health activity attempts to simply extend clinical and health education services. Practitioners and researchers are suggesting more constraining forms of intervention that aim to shape technosexuality in ways that will presumably limit the transmission of sexually transmitted infections and HIV. But a dialogical form of public health governance is desirable and possible. This dialogical form recognises how authority is shaped and reshaped, and therefore permits technosexual citizens to participate in ways that are not as easily exercised in traditional forms of public health governance. In the next concluding chapter, I will summarise these and related perspectives and reflect on relevant implications for public health and technosexuality.

8
Conclusion

The index page of *safesexpassport.com* (SSP) asked users to contemplate the idea of the eradication of sexually transmitted infections and HIV. The website offered itself as the method to do so. By directly addressing the imagination of technosexual citizens in terms of its benefits, the website referred to the transcendent qualities of technological innovation in general (Mosco, 2004) and the 'bio-technical embrace' that informs medicine in particular (Delvecchio-Good, 2001). The SSP thus established social and commercial value by offering hope for the bio-technological rationalisation of sexual interaction in a way that will eradicate disease, at least for the individual consumer. The passport metaphor also invited images of technosexual travellers of an internet-mediated world, circulating in ways free from disease and related concerns.

The example of the SSP is therefore not simply a method of avoiding sexually transmitted infections and HIV. It is an example of bio- and communication technologies combined to address technosexual citizenship. As I have noted in previous chapters, the SSP website provided instructions for gaining access to tests for HIV and sexually transmitted infections and making the results available to others through the internet. The underlying logic of the SSP was that service users will apply biological knowledge in a way that accords with public health rationalities of disease control, for example, risk avoidance. The SSP conformed to a general rationality in public health governance where the self is seen to have dominion over matters of intimacy and sexual pleasure and, accordingly, should not be instructed with regard to their sexual practice. Approaches such as these ask users to, as Rose would have it, contemplate the ethics of their actions (2001). In this view, the bio-technological eradication of HIV and sexually transmitted infections is couched, not as an instruction, but as an invitation to technosexual actors to confront their own anxieties, hopes, practices and sexual relations.

The SSP also worked to make technosexual actors visible in terms of public health rationalities. Quite literally, the mixing of internet and bio-technology is a product that can be purchased and used to view the sexual health status of prospective partners. The example of the SSP is therefore the alterity of spectacular risk. It is the opposite of the supposedly errant citizens who bareback and bug chase to transmit HIV. Technosexuality so governed is a simple system of model and errant citizens.

My interest in this book has been to reflect on such arrangements of technosexuality and public health governance. As the means for reflecting on such governance, I have developed an account of technosexual citizenship by drawing on relevant scholarship regarding sexual practice, technology and citizenship. On the basis of this conceptual framework, I addressed public health governance in three main ways: public health imperatives in connection with technosexual innovations; prevailing assumptions concerning technosexual action, with particular reference to visibility; and the bio-technological mediation of public health itself in relation to the twinned processes of medicalisation and de-medicalisation.

In the sections that follow, I want to reflect on the argument of this book with reference to key themes and perspectives. First I will consider the reflexivity implied in technosexual forms such as the questing avatar and the Viagra cyborg. I also want to make note of how these aspects of technosexuality have implications for the ethics of online intimate and sexual life. The next section considers the foundational pattern of the public health governance of technosexuality where dangers for healthy sexuality and cure are brought close together, or even superimposed. The final section makes reference to the decentring of public health and its implications. Technosexual practices appear to be implicated in configurations of authority over bio-technological knowledges and effects that may give rise to the commodification of public health.

Self-animation

Technosexuality is expressed in many ways. I have addressed only a few of these, in particular: e-dating; bio-technologies relevant for sexually transmitted infections and HIV; and their intersections. There is no doubt that other forms of technosexuality will arise which will have relevance for sexually transmitted infections and HIV, and beyond. It is difficult to characterise technosexuality because it is diverse and likely to alter. But, as I will discuss, some generalities are possible that help to reflect on the argument of this book. Whether based in bio- or communication technology, forms of technosexuality can be regarded as productively disruptive of selves, bodies and social relations. They are self-confronting in the sense that such technosexual forms are brought into existence as a matter of reflexivity. Different expressions of technosexuality can therefore be regarded as joined because they represent, more or less consciously orchestrated, self-animation of selves, bodies and relations. It is likely that such self-animation is the source of the value of technosexuality in informational capitalism. As Arvidsson has pointed out, the manner in which e-dating websites encourage e-daters to pay for their own labour is a miracle in itself (2006). Although there is dispute with regard to the reciprocal qualities of the internet in general (Holmes, 2005), it is also possible that technosexual forms in particular do not exist without an ethics of reciprocal relations.

Technosexuality is productively disruptive. As I pointed out, the term technosexual has been used to advertise a fragrance to a new niche market called into existence at the intersection of technological change and sexual desire. This observation underscores the productive nature of the relationship between technology and sexuality and how it has been colonised, or perhaps even brought into existence, by late-modern capitalism. Viagra use and and e-dating are other examples. The term technosexual also invites the prospect of the improvement of sexual experience and even sexual health. But it also raises hysterical visions of technosex monsters wreaking havoc. The notion that the internet corrodes intimate relations or that it jeopardises sexual health are examples. As Gordo-Lopez and Cleminson have noted, technosexuality can also be shown to have a genealogy in the long-standing question of governance that arises at the intersection of machinic movement, liminal space, questions of miscegenation, pleasure, and sin (2004). Gordo-Lopez and Cleminson refer to both industrial age railways and the information age internet as technologies of globalisation that also have sexual implications. In a sense then, the idea of technosexuality is already exhausted. It refers to the hopes and anxieties that, for some time, have been mobilised in and around the promise of technological modernisation.

Technosexuality is also already technosexual citizenship. The idea of questing avatars reveals the social and psychological implications of technologically-mediated experience. Technosexual actors need to bring themselves into being and negotiate intimate life, both on and through the internet and related technologies. As Turkle and many others have pointed out, such self-animation requires an engagement with oneself, with potentially productive implications for psyche and social interaction. It seems also the case that this existential challenge is too much for many of us. Technosexual forms are surprisingly conventional in the face of what has been said to be so much possibility (Slater, 1998). The cyber-ethnographies of internet-mediated intimate and sexual life have established that technosexual practices necessarily draw on an ethics of reciprocity, authenticity and transparency to deal with the social and technical challenges of making online intimate life. Such ethical considerations are most clearly expressed in the early forms of internet-based technosexuality (Marshall, 2003; Slater, 1998). It is possible to argue therefore, that the ethical considerations of technosexual life do not arise outside its practice. An ethics for the "... quotidian materiality" (Gordo-Lopez & Cleminson, 2004: 111) of online intimate life is the necessary condition for its existence. Similarly, the Viagra cyborg, based on the work of Annie Potts (Potts, 2005), draws attention to the ways in which bio-technologies are implicated in questions of sexual embodiment, the decentring of medical authority over sexual practice, and the production of patient/consumers. Viagra-use and the applications of bio-technology more generally, therefore imply a different kind of productive self-animation. In addition, the internet-based self-prescribing of Viagra exemplifies the hybridisation of bio- and communication technologies and underscores the involvement of technosexuality in the reconfiguration of authority over bio-technological knowledge and effects.

Such technosexual citizenship intersects with debates regarding ethical sexual relations in general. Indeed, technosexual practices are often found at the centre of debates regarding intimate and sexual life in late modernity where it is often subject to cultural pessimism (Weeks, 2007). Technosexuality is sometimes taken to be a reflection of moral decline or technologically-driven anomie. It may also be that attempts to govern technosexuality reinforce its status as a danger to public health because it exists outside of, or interrupts, heteronormative domesticity. In a more optimistic line of argument, it is possible to trace an arc of continuity from the reciprocal ethics that is the foundation of online intimate life, through the ethics of mutual care that has been articulated by cyber-feminism, into sexual citizenship articulated around a minimal universalism that permits the framing of questions of social justice. As Plummer has argued, this minimal universalism is not dogma, but a sensitising strategy (2003). Not surprisingly, there is a fervent and creative debate regarding sexual citizenship that takes its premises as a starting point for critical inquiry. For example, the assimilating and normalising aspects of sexual citizenship have been strenuously challenged (Richardson, 2004). Researchers who have considered citizenship in research regarding sexual heath have argued that it is indeed relevant if recognised as relational, situated and strategic (Brown, 2006; Bryant, 2006; Squire, 1999). A key argument here is that sexual citizenship, understood as a system of rights and responsibilities, can map onto various unhelpful identities, in particular, an opposition of model and errant citizens, as in the opposition of the SSP and spectacular risk. Alternatively, sexual citizenship can also be recognised as an ethics of relating figured around mutual care and cooperation. In this view, technosexual citizenship can be taken to be a critical theory for the practice of technologically-mediated intimate and sexual life, as opposed to constitutive of polarised model and errant identities.

Governing through danger/cure

As the examples I have used in this book demonstrate, public health does intervene in technosexual citizenship. But it seems that, for some of this public health governance, a central principle is that danger and cure can be the same. It is also the case that technological determinism and individualism have been relayed into some research regarding the implications of technosexuality for sexually transmitted infections and HIV. This strategy of governing via danger/cure turns on the capacity of the internet, bio-technologies, and their hybrids to make technosexuality visible, and therefore amenable to governance. Technosexuality as both dangerous and the means to a better public health, deterministic assumptions regarding technosexual action, and the panoptic exploitation of technosexuality are particularly problematic in forms of public health that are not reflexive with their own contribution to technosexuality.

Public health attention to questions of technosexuality is shaped around the binary of danger and cure, echoing the way in which technosexuality itself reflects anxiety and hope regarding technological modernisation. Unwittingly or not, this basic premise gives rise to forms of public health figured around a notion of technosexual practices as a problem for sexual health, but also as a method for extending itself. This is a compelling duality that provides a basic governmental logic for forms of public health in the area of technosexuality and beyond.

I also noted a preoccupation in public health research with young people and gay men, reflecting their prominent status as technosexual citizens and in epidemiological knowledge regarding sexually transmitted infections and HIV. But as Halperin has argued in connection with the psycho-pathologisation of the sexuality of gay men in recent HIV research (Halperin, 2007), public health governance is not just applied to technosexual practices, it helps them to come into being, by: exercising its assumptions regarding the effects of technology and sexual agency; and compelling forms of technosexuality. Practices such internet-mediated sorting of sexual partners with reference to their sexual health status are examples because they rely on both bio- and communication technology and express responses to the risk imperative of public health governance.

Research attempting to quantify the contribution of technosexuality to the risk of sexually transmitted infections and HIV draws on assumptions of technological determinism and notions of individualism. E-dating research in particular is subject to a form of determinism expressed through the idea that the anonymity of online communication is the cause of problems. The anonymity concept is based on a comparison of online and offline social life that privileges offline social interaction as authentic social experience, less available to anonymity and the corruption of truth. This privileging of offline social interaction may be misleading. It does not altogether cohere with the cyber-ethnographies of intimate online life, which argue that, while technosexual citizens appeared to be aware of questions of authenticity, reciprocity and transparency were the necessary conditions of online sociality, at least in relation to sexual and intimate life. The anonymity perspective also overlooks the ways in which prejudices regarding sexual difference shape how the truth of sexual desire is expressed in both online and offline situations. This can mean that people are able to express the 'truth' of themselves online, when they cannot so easily elsewhere (Hillier & Harrison, 2007). Research regarding HIV bio-technologies exhibits some of the same problems of e-dating research, but in addition, does not properly engage with how citizens are positioned according to blame. But all this research does suggest self-aware use of bio- and communication technologies on the part of technosexual citizens. For example, it is the case that e-dating and HIV bio-technologies are hybridised. Hybridisation is partly derived from the affinity between bio- and communication technologies in terms of how they both lend themselves to the categorisation and coding of aspects of embodiment, such as sexual health status. But more importantly, these hybrids are brought into being through the imperatives of public health governance, articulated through the self-conscious practices of individuals. In contrast with deterministic understandings of sexual practice and technology, there is a case for acknowledging the self-aware engagements with technologies and imperatives on the part of technosexual citizens. In this view, attention is paid to how people make the technologies work in light of their desires and prevailing social expectations, including those that apply to public health.

I have also made a case that technosexuality supplies an 'epistemological' strategy for public health governance. I based this notion on the visualising capacities of internet technologies, but also on the manner in which bio-technologies can be used to reveal aspects of individual embodiment. In this line of argument, it is not so much that technosexuality is a sexual health problem, but that sexual practices thought to be involved in the transmission of sexually transmitted infections and HIV, come into view in ways that were not previously available. Such visions of sexual practice help mobilise public health attention and provide the basis for intervention. This perspective underlines the dual interest of public health governance in technosexuality as a source of danger and as a means for extending itself. It also suggests why there is such a focus on technosexuality despite ambiguous evidence for sexual health concerns. The idea that anonymity is a cause of problems for public health, is, in fact, part of this exercise of using the internet and related technologies to make technosexual citizens more visible in terms of public health rationalities. The operation of this logic is most clearly expressed in the focus on spectacular forms of risk that mobilise the forensic and blaming aspects of risk culture.

It also appears that, self-consciously or not, public health governance is obliged to rely on this duality of danger/cure. I have noted how, despite conceptual problems, both e-dating and HIV bio-technologies now have a taken for granted status as problems for sexual health. The durability of these assumptions in the face of conceptual thinness can be traced back into the cultural significance of technosexuality and in particular, the way in which it mobilises the meanings of both danger and transcendence. It may also be the case therefore, that the only permissible method of addressing technosexuality as a matter of public health is via the duality of danger and cure. To address technosexuality as a matter of sexual health education or even social justice may not be acceptable for some governments and public institutions. In this regard, such governance conforms to the pattern of medicine in general. As has been long recognised, medicine itself relies on its power over the definition of pathology as the means for justifying its exercise of cure (Illich, 1975). In addition, reluctance on the part of public health to engage in alternative ways with technosexuality may be an example of a more general, longstanding reluctance on the part of public administration to directly address the private sphere of intimate and sexual life, and in particular, desire and pleasure. This feature of public health governance also indicates a tension concerning technology and desire. Public health governance attends to, and as I have argued helps bring into being, bio-technologically mediated sexual sociality. But, as the figures of the questing avatar and the Viagra cyborg suggest, technosexuality also concerns desire, pleasure and intimacy. Because public health can only be interested in imperatives regarding danger/cure, it cannot properly engage with the other possibilities of technosexual experience. In this way, public health governance is fated to provoke a cultural contest between the bio-technological rationalising of sexual sociality and the disruptively productive qualities of technosexuality that articulate desire and pleasure in intimate relations.

The passing of 'public' health

There is therefore an argument that public health governance tied to the duality of danger/cure imposes itself on a productive technosexuality. However, it may also be the case that aspects of technosexuality are influencing how public health is organised. In its pursuit of the control of the spread of diseases, public health itself is found to draw on a mix of functionalist notions of social obligation and a notional sovereign self. This mix gives public health an inchoate character and raises questions concerning how citizenship is understood, particularly in connection with bio-technological knowledge. In addition, partly through technosexuality, public health is produced in the relays and networks of multiple social actors, in which can be found a form of public health as a commodity for purchase, among other effects. Such changes underline the necessity for critical dialogue regarding public health in technologically-mediated societies.

As I have argued, altruism, contagion, risk, and forensics are all present in public health governance that addresses technosexuality. These rationalities imply different assumptions regarding self and society. However, various authors (Berridge, 1997; Valentine, 2005; Waldby et al., 2004) have argued that these forms of public health governance are being transformed through processes of bio-technologisation. The example of the SSP suggests a perfected bio-technological control of sexually trans-mitted infections and HIV, facilitated by internet-based commun-ication mixed with biological technology. However, approaches like these draw on a somewhat incoherent set of assumptions regarding self and society, and therefore give rise to paradoxical conceptualisations such as, altruism as both giving and withholding, self-protection and partner protection, and altruistic individualism. Public heath gover-nance so far has not been very clear about how such forms of subjec-tivity should be combined. Public health governance organised through this mix of functionalism and late modern notions of self, omits the guarantee of equivalence in reciprocal relations that has been consid-ered to provide the basis for sociality. Instead, public health appears to want to bring into being, citizens typed according to their biological character and responsibilities.

In addition, features of technosexuality are at the heart of the decentring of public health, and it would appear, the strengthening of consumer-provider relations. Because public health has taken up the methods of bio-technological mediation to address technosexuality, it is now thoroughly embedded in the relays and networks of multiple actors. Patients, clinicians, government, media and commercial organ-isations are all implicated in public health. This perspective draws attention to the idea that citizens do not sit outside public health, nor are they simply addressed by it. Citizens are part of the relays and net-works of social relations where they are required to bring public health into being. In addition, technosexuality gives rise to a specific configur-ation of sexual action, technology and authority, in particular: sexual pleasure as a domain of the self-determining individual; authority delim-ited by such assumptions concerning sexual practice and especially sexual pleasure; technological innovations that impinge on sexual practice; and the interests of other actors, such as those developing and marketing technologies. As the example of the SSP suggests, consumer-provider relations are coming to feature in public health governance, as in technosexuality in general. The emergence of forms of public health that draw on technosexual self-animation and reinforce consumer-provider relations create new questions for technosexual citizens and public health governance alike. For example, we are not sure how public health governance will come to be organised in bio-technologically medi-ated societies. There are signs that further complexity is likely.

Public health is thus troubled from within and without. Its foundational assumptions of self and society are found wanting and its authority over, for example sexual health, is fragmenting, partly due to technosexuality.

I want to argue that technosexual citizenship as critical theory can help address this situation. The next time you find a spam email asking you to consider some chemical or website to improve your intimate and sexual life, consider how you are being invited to become technosexual. The email will more than likely invite you to consider the prospect of a better intimate and sexual life through technosexual self-animation. But this invitation is also a significant ethical challenge to do with the question, How shall I be technosexual? The same question is posed in the SSP and other examples, but in these cases, self-confrontation concerns public health imperatives. If we wish, these ethical challenges can be extended to the question, How shall I relate technosexually? I would also like to argue that, a useful public health may be one that can reflect on itself, or at least, offer the possibility of negotiating its limitations with citizens. Perhaps the most significant challenge is finding a form of public health for technosexuality that can sustain a social justice argument with reference to sexual autonomy and also support efforts that help sexual actors to care for one another.

Bibliography

Adam, A. (2001), 'Cyberstalking: gender and computer ethics', in Green, E. and Adam, A. (eds), *Virtual gender: Technology, consumption and identity*, (London: Routledge).

Adam, B. (2005), 'Constructing the neoliberal sexual actor: responsibility and care of the self in the discourse of barebackers', *Culture, Health and Sexuality*, 7, 4, 333–346.

Adams, B. (2004), 'Intimate confessions', *HIV Plus*, www.hivplusmag.com, 8 October 2007.

Adkins, L. (2002), *Revisions: gender and sexuality in late modernity*, (Buckingham: Open University Press).

Alcorn, K. (2002), 'Ultra short-course AZT reduces mother to child transmission', *Aidsmap News*. www.aidsmap.com. Published 8 July. Accessed 15 January 2008, 15 January 2008.

Anderton, J. and Valdiserri, R. (2005), 'Combating syphilis and HIV among users of internet chatrooms', *Journal of Health Communication*, 10, 665–671.

Armstrong, D. (1993), 'From clinical gaze to regime of total health', *Health and well-being*, (London: Macmillan: Open University).

Armstrong, D. (1995), 'The rise of surveillance medicine', *Sociology of Health and Illness*, 17, 3, 393–404.

Arvidsson, A. (2006), '"Quality singles": internet dating and the work of fantasy', *New Media & Society*, 8, 4, 671–690.

Ashford, C. (2006), 'The only gay in the village: Sexuality and the net', *Information & Communication Technology Law*, 15, 3, 275–289.

Attwood, F. (2006), 'Sexed up: Theorizing the sexualisation of culture', *Sexualities*, 9, 1, 77–94.

Bass, B. (2001), 'The sexual performance perfection industry and the medicalisation of male sexuality', *The Family Journal: Counselling and Therapy for Couples and Families*, 9, 3, 337–340.

Bauman, Z. (2003), *Liquid love: on the frailty of human bonds*, (Cambridge: Polity).

Beck, U. (1992), *Risk society: towards a new modernity*, (London: Sage).

Beck, U. and Beck-Gernsheim, E. (1995), *The normal chaos of love*, (Cambridge: Polity).

Beck, U. and Beck-Gernsheim, E. (2002), *Individualisation: institutionalised individualism and its social and political consequences*, (London: Sage).

Beharrell, P. (1993), 'AIDS and the British Press', in Eldridge, J. (ed.), *Getting the Message*, (London: Routledge).

Bell, D. and Binnie, J. (2004), 'Authenticating queer space: Citizenship, urbanism and governance', *Urban Studies*, 41, 9, 1807–1820.

Ben-Ze'ev, A. (2004), *Love online: Emotions on the internet*, (Cambridge: Cambridge University Press).

Berridge, V. (1997), 'AIDS and the gift relationship in the UK', in Oakley, A. and Ashton, J. (eds), *The gift relationship: From Human blood to social policy, by Richard Titumss*, (London: LSE Books).

Beswick, T. (2000), 'Bareback "outings" spark debate over well-known secret', *Bay Area Reporter*, San Francisco, 27 July.

Bimbi, D. and Parsons, J. (2007), 'Barebacking among internet based male sex workers', in Halkitis, P., Wilton, L. and Drescher, J. (eds), *Barebacking: psychosocial and public health approaches*, (Binghamton: Haworth Medical Press).

Biressi, A. and Nunn, H. (2005), *Reality TV: realism and revelation*, (London: Wallflower Press).

Boies, S. (2002), 'University students' uses of and reactions to online sexual information and entertainment: links to online and offline sexual behaviour', *The Canadian Journal of Human Sexuality*, 11, 2, 77–89.

Bolding, G., Davis, M., Hart, G., Sherr, L. and Elford, J. (2005), 'Gay men who look for sex on the Internet: is there more HIV/STI risk with online partners?' *AIDS*, 19, 961–968.

Bordo, S. (1999), *The male body: a new look at men in public and private*, (New York: Farrar, Straus and Giroux).

Brett, S. (2006), 'Where do I get one of those house-hunks?' *The Sydney Morning Herald*, Sydney, 14 April.

Brown, M. (2006), 'Sexual citizenship, political obligation and disease ecology in gay Seattle', *Political Geography*, 25, 874–898.

Bryant, J. (2006), 'Rights, responsibilities and citizenship in heterosexual women's talk about sex: Promoting women's sexual health and safety', *Health Sociology Review*, 15, 3, 277–286.

Burke, S. (2000), 'In search of lesbian community in an electronic world', *Cyberpsychology and Behaviour*, 3, 4, 591–604.

Butler, D. and Smith, D. (2007), 'Serosorting can potentially increase HIV transmissions', *AIDS*, 21, 9, 1218–1220.

Cairns, G. (2000), 'Pleasure and risk: a barebacking manifesto', *Positive Nation*, May 2000, 16–20.

Carballo-Dieguez, A. and Bauermeister, J. (2004), '"Barebacking": intentional condomless anal sex in HIV-risk contexts. Reasons for and against it', *Journal of Homosexuality*, 47, 1, 1–16.

Carballo-Dieguez, A., Dowsett, G., Ventuneac, A., Remien, R., Balan, I., Dolevzal, C., Luciano, O. and Lin, P. (2006), 'Cybercartography of popular internet sites used by New York City men who have sex with men interested in bareback sex', *AIDS Education & Prevention*, 18, 6, 475–489.

Carter, D. (2005), 'Living in virtual communities: an ethnography of human relationships in cyberspace', *Information, Communication & Society*, 8, 2, 148–167.

Castells, M. (2000), *The information age: economy, society and culture. Volume one: the rise of network society* (Second Edition), (Malden: Blackwell).

Clatts, M., Goldsamt, L. and Yi, H. (2005), 'An emerging risk environment: a preliminary epidemiological profile of an MSM POZ Party in New York City', *Sexually Transmitted Infections*, 81, 373–376.

Cohen, D., McCubbin, M., Collin, J. and Perodeau, G. (2001), 'Medications as social phenomena', *Health*, 5, 4, 441–469.

Cole, G. (2007), 'Barebacking: transformations, dissociations and the theatre of countertransference', *Studies in Gender and Sexuality*, 8, 1, 49–68.

Connell, R. and Dowsett, G. (1999), 'The unclean motion of the generative parts: frameworks in western thought on sexuality', in Parker, R. and Aggleton, P. (eds), *Culture, society and sexuality: a reader*, (London: UCL Press/ Taylor and Francis).

Conrad, P. and Leiter, V. (2004), 'Medicalisation, markets and consumers', *Journal of Health and Social Behaviour*, 45, 158–176.

Cook, H. (2005), 'The English sexual revolution: technology and social change', *History Workshop Journal*, 59, 109–128.

Cooper, A. and Griffin-Shelley, E. (2002), 'Introduction. The Internet: the next sexual revolution', in Cooper, A. (ed.), *Sex and the Internet: A guidebook for clinicians*, (New York: Brunner-Routledge).

Cooper, A., Morahan-Martin, J., Mathy, R. and Maheu, M. (2002), 'Toward an increased understanding of user demographics in online sexual activities', *Journal of Sex & Marital Therapy*, 28, 105–129.

Cooper, A., Scherer, C., Boies, S. and Gordon, B. (1999), 'Sexuality and the Internet: from sexual exploration to pathological expression', *Professional Psychology: Research and Practice*, 30, 2, 154–164.

Cossman, B. (2002), 'Sexing citizenship, privatising sex', *Citizenship Studies*, 6, 4, 483–506.

Coveney, J. and Bunton, R. (2003), 'In pursuit of the study of pleasure: implications for health research and practice', *Health: An Interdisciplinary Journal for the Social Study of Health, Illness and Medicine*, 7, 2, 161–179.

Cox, P. (2007), 'Compulsion, voluntarism, and venereal disease: governing sexual health in England after the Contagious Diseases Act', *Journal of British Studies*, 46, 91–115.

Crawford, J., Lawless, S. and Kippax, S. (1997), 'Positive women and heterosexuality: problems of disclosure of serostatus to sexual partners', in Aggleton, P., Davies, P. and Hart, G. (eds), *AIDS, activism and alliances*, (London: Taylor & Francis).

Crimp, D. (2002), 'Melancholia and moralism: an introduction', in *Melancholia and moralism: essays on AIDS and queer politics*, (Cambridge, Massachusetts: The MIT Press).

Crossley, M. (2004), 'Making sense of "barebacking": gay men's narratives, unsafe sex and the "resistance habitus"', *British Journal of Social Psychology*, 43, 225–244.

Cullen, J. and Cohn, S. (2006), 'Making sense of mediated information: Empowerment and dependency', in Webster, A. (ed.), *New technologies in health care: Challenge, change and innovation*, (Houndmills: Palgrave).

Cusick, L. and Rhodes, T. (2000), 'Sustaining sexual safety in relationships: HIV positive people and their sexual partners', *Culture, Health and Sexuality*, 2, 4, 473–487.

Davis, M. (2002), 'HIV prevention rationalities and serostatus in the risk narratives of gay men', *Sexualities*, 5, 3, 281–299.

Davis, M. (2007), 'Identity, expertise and HIV risk in a case study of reflexivity and medical technologies', *Sociology*, 41, 6, 1003–1019.

Davis, M. (2008), 'The "loss of community" and other problems for sexual citizenship in recent HIV prevention', *Sociology of Health and Illness*, 30, 3, 182–196.

Davis, M. (in press), 'Spectacular risk, public health and the technological mediation of the sexual practices of gay men', in Broom, A. and Tovey, P. (eds), *Men's Health: Body, Identity and Social Context*, (Chichester: John Wiley & Sons).

Davis, M., Bolding, G., Hart, G., Sherr, L. and Elford, J. (2004), 'Reflecting on the experience of interviewing online: perspectives from the Internet and HIV study in London', *AIDS Care*, 16, 8, 944–952.

Davis, M., Frankis, J. and Flowers, P. (2006a), 'Uncertainty and technological horizon in qualitative interviews about HIV treatment', *Health: An Interdisciplinary Journal for the Social Study of Health, Illness and Medicine*, 10, 3, 323–344.

Davis, M., Hart, G., Bolding, G., Sherr, L. and Elford, J. (2006b), 'E-dating, identity and HIV prevention: theorising sexual interaction, risk and network society', *Sociology of Health and Illness*, 28, 4, 457–478.

Davis, M., Hart, G., Bolding, G., Sherr, L. and Elford, J. (2006c), 'Sex and the Internet: gay men, risk reduction and serostatus', *Culture, Health and Sexuality*, 8, 2, 161–174.

Davis, M., Hart, G., Imrie, J., Davidson, O., Williams, I. and Stephenson, J. (2002), '"HIV is HIV to me": meanings of treatments, viral load and reinfection among gay men with HIV', *Health, Risk and Society*, 4, 1, 31–43.

Dawson, A., Ross, M., Henry, D. and Freeman, A. (2007), 'Evidence of HIV transmission risk in barebacking Men-Who-Have-Sex-With-Men: cases from the Internet', in Halkitis, P., Wilton, L. and Drescher, J. (eds), *Barebacking: psychosocial and public health approaches*, (Binghamton: Haworth Medical Press).

Del Casino, V. (2007), 'Flaccid theory and the geographies of sexual health in the age of Viagra TM', *Health & Place*, 13, 904–911.

Delmonico, D., Griffin, E. and Carnes, P. (2002), 'Treating online compulsive sexual behaviour: When cybersex is the drug of choice', in Cooper, A. (ed.), *Sex and the Internet: A guidebook for clinicians*, (New York: Brunner-Routledge).

Delvecchio-Good, M. (2001), 'The biotechnical embrace', *Culture, Medicine and Psychiatry*, 25, 395–410.

Denzin, N. (1995), *The cinematic society: the voyeurs gaze*, (London: Sage).

Dodds, C. (2002), 'Messages of responsibility: HIV/AIDS prevention materials in England', *Health: An Interdisciplinary Journal for the Social Study of Health, Illness and Medicine*, 6, 2, 139–171.

Dodds, J., Mercey, D., Parry, J. and Johnson, A. (2004), 'Increasing risk behaviour and high levels of undiagnosed HIV infection in a community sample of homosexual men', *Sexually Transmitted Infections*, 80, 236–240.

Douglas, M. (1992), *Risk and blame: essays in cultural theory*, (London: Routledge).

Dowsett, G., Bollen, J., McInnes, D., Couch, M. and Edwards, B. (2001), 'HIV/AIDS and constructs of gay community: researching educational practice within community-based health promotion for gay men', *International Journal of Social Research Methodology*, 4, 3, 205–223.

Dowsett, G., Williams, H., Ventuneac, A. and Carballo-Dieguez, A. (2008), '"Taking it like a man": Masculinity and barebacking online', *Sexualities*, 11, 1/2, 121–141.

Elford, J. (2006), 'Changing patterns of sexual behaviour in the era of highly active antiretroviral therapy', *Current Opinion in Infectious Diseases*, 19, 26–32.

Elford, J. and Hart, G. (2005), 'HAART, viral load and sexual risk behaviour', *AIDS*, 19, 205–207.

Elford, J., Bolding, G., Sherr, L. and Hart, G. (2007), 'No evidence of an increase in serosorting with casual partners among HIV-negative gay men in London, 1998–2005', *AIDS*, 21, 2, 243–245.

Elliott, F. (2004), '"Gift" of potentially lethal sex is linked to rise in HIV cases', *The Independent*, 18 April.

Ellis, A., Highleyman, L., Schaub, K. and White, M. (2002), *The Harvey Milk Institute guide to Lesbian, Gay, Bisexual, Transgender, and Queer Internet Research*, (New York: Harrington Park Press).

Epstein, S. (ed.) (1996), *Impure science: AIDS, activism and the politics of knowledge*, University of California Press, Berkeley.

Epstein, S. (2000), 'Whose identities, which differences? Activism and the changing terrain of biomedicalisation', *Paper presented at HIV and Related Diseases Conference (HARD) Social Research Conference, Gazebo Hotel, Sydney, May 13, 2000*.

Epstein, S. (2003), 'Sexualising governance and medicalising identities: the emergence of "state-centred" LGBT health politics in the United States', *Sexualities*, 6, 2, 131–171.

Etiebet, M., Fransman, D., Forsyth, B., Coetzee, N. and Hussey, G. (2004), 'Integrating prevention of mother-to-child HIV transmission into antenatal care: learning from the experiences of women in South Africa', *AIDS Care*, 16, 1, 37–46.

Ettorre, E., Rothman, B. and Steinberg, D. (2006), 'Feminism confronts the genome: introduction', *New Genetics and Society*, 25, 2, 133–142.

Fisher, D., Malow, R., Rosenberg, R., Reynolds, G., Farerell, N. and Jaffe, A. (2006), 'Recreational Viagra use and sexual risk among drug abusing men', *American Journal of Infectious Diseases*, 2, 2, 107–114.

Fisher, W. and Barak, A. (2001), 'Internet pornography: a social psychological perspective on Internet sexuality', *Journal of Sex Research*, 38, 4, 312–323.

Flowers, P. (2001), 'Gay men and HIV/AIDS risk management', *Health*, 5, 50–75.

Flowers, P. and Langdridge, D. (2007), 'Offending the other: Deconstructing narratives of deviance and pathology', *British Journal of Social Psychology*, 46, 3, 679–690.

Flowers, P., Smith, J., Sheeran, P. and Beail, N. (1997), 'Health and romance: understanding unprotected sex in relationships between gay men', *British Journal of Health Psychology*, 2, 73–86.

Foucault, M. (1976), *The birth of the clinic: an archaeology of medical perception*, (London: Tavistock Publications).

Foucault, M. (1982), *Discipline and punish: the birth of the prison*, (Harmondsworth: Penguin).

Fox, N. and Ward, K. (2006), 'Health identities: from expert patient to resisting consumer', *Health: An Interdisciplinary Journal for the Social Study of Health, Illness and Medicine*, 10, 4, 461–479.

Freeman, G. (2003), 'In search of death: Bug chasers: the men who long to be HIV+', *Rolling Stone*, Digital edition: www.rollingstone.com. Published 23 January. Accessed 14 August 2007.

Garland, E. (2004), 'Reinventing sex: new technologies and changing attitudes', *The Futurist*, November–December 2004, 41–46.

Gauthier, D. and Forsyth, C. (1999), 'Bareback sex, bug chasers and the gift of death', *Deviant Behaviour*, 20, 85–100.

Gazzard, B. (2005), 'British HIV Association (BHIVA) guidelines for the treatment of HIV-infected adults with antiretroviral therapy (2005)', *HIV Medicine*, 6, Supplement 2, 1–61.

Gendin, S. (1999), 'Both sides now: Stephen Gendin', www.thebody.com/poz/inside/11_99/sides_gendin.htm, POZ.

Giddens, A. (1990), *The consequences of modernity*, (Cambridge: Polity).

Giddens, A. (1991), *Modernity and self identity: self and society in the late modern age*, (London: Polity).

Giddens, A. (1992), *The transformation of intimacy: sexuality, love and eroticism in modern societies*, (Cambridge: Polity).

Gilbert, L., Temby, J. and Rogers, S. (2005), 'Evaluating a teen STD prevention web site', *Journal of Adolescent Health*, 37, 236–242.

Golden, M., Wood, R., Buskin, S., Fleming, M. and Harrington, R. (2007), 'Ongoing risk behaviour among persons with HIV in medical care', *AIDS & Behaviour*, 11, 726–735.

Gordo-Lopez, A. and Cleminson, R. (2004), *Techno-sexual landscapes: Changing relations between technology and sexuality*, (London: Free Association Books).

Gosine, A. (2007), 'Brown to blonde at Gay.com: passing white in queer cyberspace', in O'Riordan and Phillips, D. (eds), *Queer online: Media, technology & sexuality*, (New York: Peter Lang).

Granzow, K. (2007), 'De-constructing "choice": The social imperative and women's use of the birth control pill', *Culture, Health & Sexuality*, 9, 1, 43–54.

Graydon, M. (2007), 'Don't bother to wrap it: Online Giftgiver and Bugchaser newsgroups, the social impact of gift exchanges and the "carnivalesque"', *Culture, Health & Sexuality*, 9, 3, 277–292.

Greco, M. (2004), 'The politics of indeterminacy and the right to health', *Theory, Culture and Society*, 21, 6, 1–22.

Green, E., Griffiths, F., Henwood, F. and Wyatt, F. (2006), 'Desperately seeking certainty: Bone densitometry, the internet and health care contexts', in Webster, A. (ed.), *New technologies in health care: Challenge, change and innovation*, (Houndmills: Palgrave).

Green, G. and Smith, R. (2004), 'The psychosocial and health care needs of HIV-positive people in the United Kingdom following HAART: a review', *HIV Medicine*, 5, Supplement 1, 1–46.

Green, G. and Sobo, E. (2000), *The endangered self: managing the social risks of HIV*, (London: Routledge).

Greenwood, H. (2007), 'His for her, hers for his', *The Sydney Morning Herald*, Sydney, Online source, 7 June 2007.

Grov, C. (2004), '"Make me your death slave": men who have sex with men and use the Internet to intentionally spread HIV', *Deviant Behaviour*, 25, 4, 329–349.

Grov, C. (2006), 'Barebacking websites: electronic environments for reducing or inducing HIV risk', *AIDS Care*, 18, 8, 990–997.

Grov, C. and Parsons, J. (2006), 'Bug chasing and gift giving: The potential for HIV transmission among barebackers on the internet', *AIDS Education and Prevention*, 18, 6, 490–503.

Grov, C., DeBusk, J., Bimbi, D., Golub, S., Nanin, J. and Parsons, J. (2007), 'Barebacking, the Internet, and harm reduction: An intercept survey with gay and bisexual men in Los Angeles and New York City', *AIDS & Behaviour*, 11, 527–536.

Halkitis, P. and Green, K. (2007), 'Sildenafil (Viagra) and club drug use in gay and bisexual men: The role of drug combinations and context', *American Journal of Men's Health*, 1, 2, 139–147.

Halkitis, P., Wilton, L. and Galatowitsch, P. (2007), 'What's in a term? How gay and bisexual men understand barebacking', in Halkitis, P., Wilton, L. and Drescher, J. (eds), *Barebacking: psychosocial and public health approaches*, (Binghamton: Haworth Medical Press).

Halperin, D. (2007), *What do gay men want? An essay on sex, risk, and subjectivity*, (Ann Arbor: The University of Michigan Press).

Haraway, D. (1991), *Simians, cyborgs and women: The reinvention of nature*, (London: Free Association).

Hardey, M. (1999), 'Doctor in the house: the Internet as a source of lay health knowledge and the challenge to expertise', *Sociology of Health and Illness*, 21, 6, 820–835.

Hardey, M. (2004), 'Mediated relationships: authenticity and the possibility of romance', *Information, Communication and Society*, 7, 2, 207–222.

Hart, G. and Wellings, K. (2002), 'Sexual behaviour and its medicalisation: in sickness and in health', *British Medical Journal*, 324, 896–900.

Hartley, H. (2006), 'The "pinking" of viagra culture: Drug industry efforts to create and repackage sex drugs for women', *Sexualities*, 9, 3, 363–378.

Harvey, K., Brown, B., Crawford, P., Macfarlane, A. and McPherson, A. (2007), '"Am I normal?" Teenagers, sexual health and the Internet', *Social Science & Medicine*, 65, 4, 771–781.

Heaphy, B. (1996), 'Medicalisation and identity formation: identity and strategy in the context of AIDS and HIV', in Weeks, J. and Holland, J. (eds), *Sexual Cultures*, (Houndmills: Macmillan).

Hearn, J. (2006), 'The implications of information and communication technologies for sexualities and sexualised violences: contradictions of sexual citizenships', *Political Geography*, 25, 8, 944–963.

Henwood, F., Wyatt, S., Hart, A. and Smith, J. (2003), '"Ignorance is bliss sometimes": constraints on the emergence of the "informed patient" in the changing landscapes of health information', *Sociology of Health & Illness*, 25, 6, 589–607.

Herdt, G. (2001), 'Stigma and the ethnographic study of HIV: problems and prospects', *AIDS and Behaviour*, 5, 2, 141–149.

Hertlain, K. and Piercy, F. (2006), 'Internet infidelity: A critical review of the literature', *The Family Journal*, 14, 4, 366–371.

Hillier, L. and Harrison, L. (2007), 'Building realities less limited than their own: young people practising same-sex attraction on the Internet', *Sexualities*, 10, 1, 82–100.

Holmes, D. (2005), *Communication theory: Media, technology, society*, (London: Sage).

Holmes, D. and Warner, D. (2005), 'The anatomy of a forbidden desire: men, penetration and semen exchange', *Nursing Inquiry*, 12, 1, 10–20.

Holmes, D., O'Byrne, P. and Gastaldo, D. (2006), 'Raw sex as limit experience: a Foucauldian analysis of unsafe anal sex between men', *Social Theory & Health*, 4, 4, 319–333.

Holt, M. and Stephenson, N. (2006), 'Living with HIV and negotiating psychological discourse', *Health: An Interdisciplinary Journal for the Social Study of Health, Illness and Medicine*, 10, 2, 211–231.

Holzemer, W. (1997), 'Living with AIDS post Vancouver', *Qualitative Health Research*, 7, 1, 5–8.

Horin, A. (2007), 'Torn apart by cyber-porn', *The Age*, Melbourne, Insight, Page 3, 26 May 2007.

Huebner, D. (2006), 'Do gay and bisexual men share researchers definitions of barebacking?', *Journal of Psychology & Human Sexuality*, 18, 1, 67–77.

Hurley, M. (2003), 'Then and now: Gay men and HIV. Monograph Series Number 46', Melbourne, Australian Research Centre in Sex, Health and Society, La Trobe University.

Illich, I. (1975), *Medical nemesis: the expropriation of health*, (Lothian Publishing).

Imrie, J., Elford, J., Kippax, S. and Hart, G. (2007), 'Biomedical HIV prevention and social science', *The Lancet*, 370, July 7, 10–11.

Jamieson, L. (2003), 'The couple: intimate and equal?' in Weeks, J., Holland, J. and Waites, M. (ed.), *Sexualities and society: a reader*, (Cambridge: Polity).

Janssen, R., Holtgrave, D., Valdiserri, R., Shepherd, M., Gayle, H. and De Cock, K. (2001), 'The serostatus approach to fighting the HIV epidemic: prevention strategies for infected individuals', *American Journal of Public Health*, 91, 7, 1019–1024.

Joglekar, N., Joshi, S., Kakde, M., Fang, G., Cianciola, M., Reynolds, S., Mehendale, S. and The HIV Prevention Trial Network Protocol Team (2007), 'Acceptability of PRO2000 vaginal gel among HIV un-infected women in Pune, India', *AIDS Care*, 19, 6, 817–821.

Jordan, T. (1999), *Cyberpower: the culture and politics of cyberspace and the Internet*, (London: Routledge).

Kaler, A. (2004), 'The future of female-controlled barrier methods for HIV prevention: female condoms', *Culture, Health & Sexuality*, 6, 6, 501–516.

Kalichman, S., Greenberg, J. and Abel, G. (1997), 'HIV-seropositive men who engage in high-risk sexual behaviour: psychological characteristics and implications for prevention', *AIDS Care*, 8, 4, 441–450.

Kelly, J., Hoffman, R., Rompa, D. and Gray, M. (1998), 'Protease inhibitor combination therapies and perceptions of gay men regarding AIDS severity and the need to maintain safer sex', *AIDS*, 12, F91–F95.

Kennedy, S. (2006), 'They're peddling death', *The Advocate*, Digital Edition, www.advocate.com, Accessed: 14 August 2007.

Keogh, P., Beardsell, S., Hickson, F. and Reid, D. (1995), 'The sexual health needs of HIV positive gay and bisexual men', London, Sigma Research & Camden and Islington Community Health Services NHS Trust, Health Promotion Service.

Keogh, P., Weatherburn, P. and Stephens, M. (1999), 'Relative safety: risk and unprotected anal intercourse among gay men diagnosed with HIV', London, Sigma Research.

King-Spooner, S. (1999), 'HIV prevention and the positive population', *International Journal of STD and AIDS*, 10, 141–150.

Kippax, S. (1999), 'Taking medicine in(to) an HIV prevention framework: renewing the importance of the new public health', *Plenary presentation at the 10th Conference on Social Aspects of AIDS, South Bank University, London, June 1999*.

Kippax, S. and Race, K. (2003), 'Sustaining safe practice: twenty years on', *Social Science and Medicine*, 57, 1–12.

Kippax, S., Crawford, J., Davis, M., Rodden, P. & Dowsett, G. (1993), 'Sustaining safe sex: a longitudinal study of a sample of homosexual men', *AIDS*, 7, 23, 257–263.

Korner, H., Hendry, O. and Kippax, S. (2006), 'Safe sex after post-exposure prophylaxis for HIV: Intentions, challenges and ambivalences in narratives of gay men', *AIDS Care*, 18, 8, 879–887.

Lather, P. (1995), 'The validity of angels: interpretive and textual strategies in researching the lives of women with HIV/AIDS', *Qualitative Inquiry*, 1, 1, 41–68.

Lawless, S., Kippax, S. and Crawford, J. (1996), 'Dirty, diseased and undeserving: the positioning of HIV positive women', *Social Science and Medicine*, 43, 9, 1371–1377.

Laza, M. (2003), 'Bug chasing', *The Mail on Sunday*, London, Review, 60–61, 2 February 2003.

Lee, H. (2007), 'Why sexual health promotion misses its audience: men who have sex with men reading texts', *Journal of Health, Organization and Management*, 21, 2, 205–219.

Levine, D. and Klausner, J. (2005), 'Lessons learned from tobacco control: A proposal for public health policy initiatives to reduce the consequences of high-risk sexual behaviour among men who have sex with men and use the internet', *Sexuality Research & Social Policy*, 2, 1, 51–58.

Liguori, A. and Lamas, M. (2003), 'Gender, sexual citizenship and HIV/AIDS', *Culture, Health & Sexuality*, 5, 1, 87–90.

Long, L. (2004), 'Anthropological perspectives on the trafficking of women for sexual exploitation', *International Migration*, 42, 1, 5–31.

Lou, C., Zhao, Q., Gao, E. and Shah, I. (2006), 'Can the Internet be used effectively to provide sex education to young people in China?' *Journal of Adolescent Health*, 39, 5, 720–728.

Lupton, D. (1995), 'Communicating health: the mass media and advertising in health promotion', in Lupton, D. (ed.), *The imperative of health*, (London: Sage).

Lupton, D. (1995), 'The embodied computer/user', *Body & Society*, 1, 3–4, 97–112.

Lupton, D. (1998), 'The end of AIDS?: AIDS reporting in the Australian press in the mid-1990s', *Critical Public Health*, 8, 1, 33–46.

Lupton, D. (1999), *Risk*, (London: Routledge).

Lupton, D. (1999a), 'Archetypes of infection: people with HIV/AIDS in the Australian press in the mid 1990s', *Sociology of Health and Illness*, 21, 1, 37–53.

Lupton, D. and Tulloch, J. (2002a), '"Life would be pretty dull without risk": voluntary risk-taking and its pleasures', *Health, Risk and Society*, 4, 2, 113–124.

Lupton, D. and Tulloch, J. (2002b), '"Risk is part of your life": risk epistemologies among a group of Australians', *Sociology*, 36, 2, 317–334.

Maguire, M. (2000), 'Bare-back sex', *Axiom*, 40, 53–54.

Mansergh, G., Marks, G., Colfax, G., Guzman, R., Rader, M. and Buchbinder, S. (2002), '"Barebacking" in a diverse sample of men who have sex with men', *AIDS*, 16, 653–659.

Mansergh, G., Shouse, R., Marks, G., Guzman, R., Rader, M., Buchbinder, S. and Colfax, G. (2006), 'Methamphetamine and sildenafil (Viagra) use are linked to unprotected receptive and insertive anal sex, respectively, in a sample of men who have sex with men', *Sexually Transmitted Infections*, 82, 131–134.

Mao, L., Crawford, J., Hospers, H., Prestage, G., Grulich, A., Kaldor, J. and Kippax, S. (2006), '"Serosorting" in casual anal sex of HIV-negative gay men is noteworthy and is increasing in Sydney, Australia', *AIDS*, 20, 8, 1204–1206.

Marcuse, H. (1972 [1964]), *One-dimensional man: Studies in the ideology of advanced industrial society*, (Boston: Beacon Press).

Marks, G., Burris, S. and Peterman, T. (1999), 'Reducing sexual transmission of HIV from those who know they are infected: the need for personal and collective responsibility', *AIDS*, 13, 297–306.

Marshall, B. (2002), '"Hard science": gendered constructions of sexual dysfunction in the "Viagra Age"', *Sexualities*, 5, 2, 131–158.

Marshall, B. (2007), 'Climacteric Redux? (Re)medicalizing the male menopause', *Men and Masculinities*, 9, 4, 509–529.

Marshall, J. (2003), 'The sexual life of cyber-savants', *The Australian Journal of Anthropology*, 14, 2, 229–248.

Mauss, M. (1990 [1950]), *The gift: The form and reason for exchange in archaic societies*, (London: Routledge).

McFarlane, M., Bull, S. and Rietmeijer, C. (2002), 'Young adults on the internet: risk behaviours for sexually transmitted diseases and HIV', *Journal of Adolescent Health*, 31, 11–16.

McFarlane, M., Kachur, R., Bull, S. and Rietmeijer, C. (2004), 'Women, the Internet, and sexually transmitted infections', *Journal of Women's Health*, 13, 6, 689–694.

McGhee, D. (2004), 'Beyond toleration: privacy, citizenship and sexual minorities in England and Wales', *The British Journal of Sociology*, 55, 3, 357–375.

McLelland, M. (2002), 'Virtual ethnography: using the Internet to study gay culture in Japan', *Sexualities*, 5, 4, 387–406.

Mitchell, J., Reid-Walsh, J. and Pithouse, K. (2004), '"And what are you reading, Miss? Oh, it is only a website": The new media and the pedagogical possibilities of digital culture as a South African "Teen Guide" to HIV/AIDS ad STDs', *Convergence: The International Journal of Research into New Media Technologies*, 10, 80–92.

Mitra, A. and Cohen, E. (1999), 'Analyzing the web: directions and challenges', in Jones, S. (ed.), *Doing Internet Research: critical issues and methods for examining the net*, (Thousand Oaks: Sage).

Mohammed, S. and Thombre, A. (2005), 'HIV/AIDS stories on the World Wide Web and transformation perspectives', *Journal of Health Communication*, 10, 347–360.

Moore, L. and Durkin, H. (2006), 'The leaky male body: forensics and the construction of the sexual suspect', in Rosenfeld, D. and Faircloth, C. (eds), *Medicalised masculinities*, (Philadelphia: Temple University Press).

Mosco, V. (2004), 'Myth and cyberspace', *The digital sublime: myth, power, and cyberspace*, (Cambridge, MA: MIT Press).

Moskowitz, D. and Roloff, M. (2007), 'The existence of a bug chasing culture', *Culture, Health & Sexuality*, 9, 4, 347–357.

Murphy, D., Rawstorne, P., Holt, M. and Ryan, D. (2004), 'Cruising and connecting online: the use of Internet chat sites by gay men in Sydney and Melbourne', Sydney, National Centre in HIV Social Research, Faculty of Arts and Social Sciences, The University of New South Wales.

Nettleton, S. and Bunton, R. (1995), 'Sociological critiques of health promotion', in Bunton, R., Nettleton, S. and Burrows, R. (eds), *The sociology of health promotion*, (London: Routledge).

Nettleton, S. and Hanlon, G. (2006), '"Pathways to the doctor" in the information age: the role of ICTs in contemporary lay referral systems', in Webster, A. (ed.), *New technologies in health care: Challenge, change and innovation*, (Houndmills: Palgrave).

Noar, S., Clark, A., Cole, C. and Lustria, M. (2006), 'Review of interactive safer sex web sites: Practice and potential', *Health Communication*, 20, 3, 233–241.

Nodin, N., Carballo-Dieguez, A., Ventuneac, A., Balan, I. and Remien, R. (2008), 'Knowledge and acceptability of alternative HIV prevention bio-medical products among MSM who bareback', *AIDS Care*, 20, 1, 106–115.

Novas, C. and Rose, N. (2000), 'Genetic risk and the birth of the somatic individual', *Economy and Society*, 29, 4, 485–513.

Nuffield-Council-on-Bioethics (2007), 'Public health: ethical issues', London, Nuffield Council on Bioethics.

Osmond, D., Pollack, L., Paul, J. and Catania, J. (2007), 'Changes in prevalence of HIV infection and sexual risk behaviour in men who have sex with men in San Francisco: 1997–2002', *American Journal of Public Health*, 97, 9, 1677–1683.

Padgett, P. (2007), 'Personal safety and sexual safety for women using online personal ads', *Sexuality Research & Social Policy*, 4, 2, 27–37.

Palandri, M. and Green, L. (2000), 'Image management in a bondage, discipline, sadomasochist subculture: a cyber-ethnography', *Cyberpsychology and Behaviour*, 3, 4, 631–641.

Parisi, L. (2004), *Abstract sex: philosophy, bio-technology and the mutations of desire*, (London: Continuum).

Parker, R. (2007), 'Sexuality, health, and human rights', *American Journal of Public Health*, 97, 6, 972–973.

Parker, R. and Aggleton, P. (2003), 'HIV and AIDS-related stigma and discrimination: a conceptual framework and implications for action', *Social Science and Medicine*, 57, 13–24.

Parsons, J., Bimbi, D. and Halkitis, P. (2002), 'Sexual compulsivity among gay/bisexual male escorts who advertise on the Internet', *Sexual Addiction and Compulsivity*, 8, 2, 101–112.

Patel, P., Taylor, M., Montoya, J., Hamburger, M., Kerndt, P. and Holmberg, S. (2006), 'Circuit parties: Sexual behaviours and HIV disclosure practices among men who have sex with men at the White Party, Palm Springs, California, 2003', *AIDS Care*, 18, 8, 1046–1049.

Peretti-Watel, P., Spire, B., Schiltz, M., Bouhnik, A., Heard, I., Lert, F., Obadia, Y. and The-VESPA-Group (2006), 'Vulnerability, unsafe sex and non-adherence to HAART: Evidence from a large sample of French HIV/AIDS outpatients', *Social Science & Medicine*, 62, 2420–2433.

Persson, A. and Newman, C. (2008), 'Making monsters: heterosexuality, crime and race in recent Western media coverage of HIV', *Sociology of Health & Illness*, 30, 4, 632–646.

Persson, A., Race, K. and Wakeford, E. (2003), 'HIV health in context: negotiating medical technology and lived experience', *Health: An Interdisciplinary Journal for the Social Study of Health, Illness and Medicine*, 7, 4, 397–415.

Petersen, A. (1996), 'Risk and the regulated self: discourse of health promotion as politics of uncertainty', *Australian and New Zealand Journal of Sociology*, 32, 1, 44–57.

Petersen, A. and Lupton, D. (1996), *The new public health: Health and self in the age of risk*, (St Leonards: Allen & Unwin).

Phillips, D. (2002), 'Negotiating the digital closet: online pseudonymity and the politics of sexual identity', *Information, Communication & Society*, 5, 3, 406–424.

Philips, F. and Morrissey, G. (2004), 'Cyberstalking and cyberpredators: A threat to safe sexuality on the internet', *Convergence: The International Journal of Research into New Media Technologies*, 10, 66–79.

Phua, V., Hopper, J. and Vazquez, O. (2002), 'Men's concerns with sex and health in personal advertisements', *Culture, Health & Sexuality*, 4, 3, 355–363.

Pillsbury, B. and Mayer, D. (2005), 'Women Connect! Strengthening communications to meet sexual and reproductive health challenges', *Journal of Health Communication*, 10, 361–371.

Plummer, K. (1995), *Telling sexual stories: power, change and social worlds*, (London: Routledge).

Plummer, K. (2003), *Intimate citizenship: private decisions and public dialogues*, (Seattle: University of Washington Press).

Poppen, P., Reisen, C., Zea, M., Bianchi, F. and Echeverry, J. (2005), 'Serostatus disclosure, seroconcordance, partner relationship, and unprotected anal intercourse among HIV-positive Latino men who have sex with men', *AIDS Education & Prevention*, 17, 3, 227–237.

Porco, T., Martin, J., Page-Shafer, K., Cheng, A., Charlebois, E., Grant, R. and Osmond, D. (2004), 'Decline in HIV infectivity following the introduction of highly active antiretroviral therapy', *AIDS*, 18, 81–88.

Potts, A. (2004), 'Deleuze on Viagra (Or, What can a "Viagra-body" do?)', *Body & Society*, 10, 1, 17–36.

Potts, A. (2005), 'Cyborg masculinity in the Viagra era', *Sexualities, Education and Gender*, 7, 1, 3–16.

Potts, A. and Tiefer, L. (2006), 'Special issue on "Viagra Culture": Introduction', *Sexualities*, 9, 3, 267–272.

Potts, A., Grace, V., Gavey, N. and Vares, T. (2004), '"Viagra stories": challenging "erectile dysfunction"', *Social Science & Medicine*, 59, 489–499.

Potts, A., Grace, V., Vares, T. and Gavey, N. (2006), '"Sex for life"? Men's counter-stories on "erectile dysfunction", male sexuality and ageing', *Sociology of Health & Illness*, 28, 3, 306–329.

Pozniak, A., Gazzard, B., Babiker, A., Churchill, D., Collins, S., Deutsch, J., Fisher, M., Johnson, M., Khoo, S., Loveday, C., Main, J., Matthews, G., Moyle, G., Nelson, M., Peters, B., Phillips, A., Pillay, D., Poppa, A., Taylor, C., Williams, I. and Youle, M. (2001), 'British HIV Association (BHIVA) guidelines for the treatment of HIV-infected adults with antiretroviral therapy', London, BHIVA.

Prestage, G., Mao, L., Fogarty, A., Van de Ven, P., Kippax, S., Crawford, J., Rawstorne, P., Kaldor, J., Jin, F. and Grulich, A. (2005), 'How has the sexual behaviour of gay men changed since the onset of AIDS: 1986–2003', *Australian and New Zealand Journal of Public Health*, 29, 6, 530–535.

Pryce, A. (2008), 'Constructing virtual selves: men, risk and the rehearsal of sexual identities and scripts in cyber chatrooms', in Petersen, A. and Wilkinson, I. (eds), *Health, risk and vulnerability*, (London: Routledge).

Purdy, L. (2001), 'Medicalisation, medical necessity, and feminist medicine', *Bioethics*, 15, 3, 248–261.

Race, K. (2001), 'The undetectable crisis: changing technologies of risk', *Sexualities*, 4, 2, 167–189.

Race, K. (2003), 'Revaluation of risk among gay men', *AIDS Education and Prevention*, 15, 4, 369–381.

Reddy, G. (2005), 'Geographies of contagion: Hijras, kothis, and the politics of sexual marginality in Hyderabad', *Anthropology & Medicine*, 12, 3, 255–270.

Reid, D., Weatherburn, P., Hickson, F. and Stephens, M. (2002), 'Know the score: findings from the National Gay Men's Sex Survey, 2001', London, Sigma Research, Faculty of Humanities and Social Sciences, University of Portsmouth.

Rhodes, S. (2004), 'Hookups or health promotion? An exploratory study of a chat room-based HIV prevention intervention for men who have sex with men', *AIDS Education and Prevention*, 16, 4, 315–327.

Rhodes, T. and Cusick, L. (2000), 'Love and intimacy in relationship management: HIV positive people and their sexual partners', *Sociology of Health and
Illness*, 22, 1, 1–26.

Richardson, D. (2004), 'Locating sexualities: From here to normality', *Sexualities*
7, 4, 391–411.

Ridge, D. (2004), '"It was an incredible thrill": the social meanings and dynam-
ics of younger gay men's experiences of barebacking in Melbourne',
Sexualities, 7, 3, 259–279.

Rietmeijer, C. and Shamos, S. (2007), 'HIV and sexually transmitted infection
prevention online: Current state and future prospects', *Sexuality Research &
Social Policy*, 4, 2, 65–73.

Rietmeijer, C., Bull, S., McFarlane, M., Patnaik, J. and Douglas, J. (2003), 'Risks
and benefits of the internet for populations at risk for sexually transmitted
infections (STIs): results from an STI clinic survey', *Sexually Transmitted
Diseases*, 30, 1, 15–19.

Riggs, D. (2006), '"Serosameness" or "serodifference"? Resisting polarised discourse of identity and relationality in the context of HIV', *Sexualities*, 9, 4,
409–422.

Rofes, E. (1998), *Dry bones breathe: gay men creating post-AIDS identities and cultures*, (New York: Harrington Park Press).

Rofes, E. (1999), 'Barebacking and the new AIDS hysteria', web, www.manag-
ingdesire.org/sexpanic/rofes499.html.

Rose, N. (2001), 'The politics of life itself', *Theory, Culture and Society*, 18, 6,
1–30.

Rosenfeld, D. and Faircloth, C. (2006), 'Introduction: Medicalised masculinities:
The missing link?' in Rosenfeld, D. and Faircloth, C. (eds), *Medicalised masculinities*, (Philadelphia: Temple University Press).

Rosengarten, M. (2004), 'Consumer activism in the pharmacology of HIV', *Body
& Society*, 10, 1, 91–107.

Rosengarten, M., Race, K. and Kippax, S. (2001), '"Touch wood, everything will
be OK": gay men's understandings of clinical markers in sexual practice',
Sydney, National Centre in HIV Social Research.

Rosenstock, I. (1974), 'Historical origins of the Health Belief Model', *Health
Education Monographs*, 2, 4, 328–335.

Ross, M., Rosser, B., Coleman, E. and Mazin, R. (2006), 'Misrepresentation on
the internet and in real life about sex and HIV: a study of Latino men who
have sex with men', *Culture, Health & Sexuality*, 8, 2, 133–144.

Salomon, H., Wainberg, M., Brenner, B., Quan, Y., Rouleau, D., Cote, P.,
LeBlanc, R., Lefebvre, E., Spira, B., Tsoukas, C., Sekaly, R., Conway, B., Mayers,
D., Routy, J. and Investigators-of-the-Quebec-Primary-Infection-Study (2000),
'Prevalence of HIV-1 resistant to antiretroviral drugs in 81 individuals newly
infected by sexual contact or injecting drug use', *AIDS*, 14, F17–F23.

Sanders, T. (2005), 'Researching the online sex work community', in Hine, C.
(ed.), *Virtual methods: issues in social research on the internet*, (Oxford: Berg).

Scarce, M. (1999), 'A ride on the wild side', *POZ*, February.

Shapiro, K. and Ray, S. (2007), 'Sexual health for people living with HIV',
Reproductive Health Matters, 15, 29 Supplement, 67–92.

Sheon, N. and Crosby, M. (2004), 'Ambivalent tales of HIV disclosure in San
Francisco', *Social Science and Medicine*, 58, 2105–2118.

Shernoff, M. (2006), 'Condomless sex: gay men, barebacking and harm reduction', *Social Work*, 51, 2, 106–113.

Sherr, L., Bolding, G., Elford, J. and Maguire, M. (2000), 'Viagra use and sexual risk behaviour among gay men in London', *AIDS*, 14, 13, 8.

Signorile, M. (1997), 'Bareback and restless', OUT, July. http://www.signorile.com/articles/outbbr.html.

Slater, D. (1998), 'Trading sexpics on IRC: embodiment and authenticity on the Internet', *Body & Society*, 4, 4, 91–117.

Slater, D. (2002), 'Making things real: ethics and order on the Internet', *Theory, Culture & Society*, 19, 5/6, 227–245.

Slavin, S., Batrouney, C. and Murphy, D. (2007), 'Fear appeals and treatment side-effects: An effective combination for HIV prevention?' *AIDS Care*, 19, 1, 130–137.

Smaill, B. (2004), 'Online personals and narratives of the self: Australia's RSVP', *Convergence: The International Journal of Research into New Media Technologies*, 10, 93–107.

Small, N. (1996), 'Intimacy, altruism and the loneliness of moral choice: the case of HIV positive health workers', in Weeks, J. and Holland, J. (eds), *Sexual Cultures*, (Houndmills: Macmillan).

Sontag, S. (1988), *AIDS and its metaphors*, (London: Penguin).

Spindler, H., Scheer, S., Chen, S., Klausner, J., Katz, M., Valleroy, L. and Schwarcz, S. (2007), 'Viagra, methamphetamine, and HIV risk: Results from a probability sample of MSM, San Francisco', *Sexually Transmitted Diseases*, 34, 8, 586–591.

Springer, C. (1996), *Electronic eros: bodies and desire in the postindustrial age*, (Austin: University of Texas Press).

Squire, C. (1999), '"Neighbours who might become friends": selves, genre and citizenship in narratives of HIV', *The Sociological Quarterly*, 40, 1, 109–138.

Stevenson, F. and Scambler, G. (2005), 'The relationship between medicine and the public: the challenge of "concordance"', *Health*, 9, 1, 5–21.

Stokes, C. (2007), 'Representin' in cyberspace: Sexual scripts, self-definition, and hip hop culture in Black America adolescent girls' home pages', *Culture, Health & Sexuality*, 9, 2, 169–184.

Suarez, T. and Miller, J. (2001), 'Negotiating risks in context: a perspective on unprotected anal intercourse and barebacking among men who have sex with men – where do we go from here?' *Archives of Sexual Behaviour*, 30, 3, 287–300.

Tewksbury, R. (2003), 'Bareback sex and the quest for HIV: assessing the relationship in Internet personal advertisements of men who have sex with men', *Deviant Behaviour*, 24, 5, 467–482.

Tewksbury, R. (2006), '"Click here for HIV": an analysis of Internet-based bug chasers and bug givers', *Deviant Behaviour*, 27, 4, 379–395.

Thomas, A., Ross, M. and Harris, K. (2007), 'Coming out online: Interpretations of young men's stories', *Sexuality Research & Social Policy*, 4, 2, 5–17.

Tiefer, L. (2006), 'The Viagra phenomenon', *Sexualities*, 9, 3, 273–294.

Titmuss, R. (1970), *The gift relationship: From human blood to social policy*, (London: George Allen & Unwin).

Tomlinson, J. (1999), *Globalisation and culture*, (Cambridge: Polity).

Treichler, P. (1999), *How to have theory in an epidemic: cultural chronicles of AIDS*, (Durham: Duke University Press).

Triffitt, K. and People Living With HIV/AIDS NSW (2004), 'Let's talk about it: me, you and sex', Sydney, People Living with HIV/AIDS, New South Wales.

Turkle, S. (1997 [1995]), *Life on the screen: identity in the age of the Internet*, (London: Phoenix).

Turkle, S. (1999), 'Cyberspace and identity', *Contemporary Sociology*, 28, 6, 643–648.

Valentine, K. (2005), 'Citizenship, identity, blood donation', *Body & Society*, 11, 2, 113–128.

van Campenhoudt, L. (1999), 'The relational rationality of risk and uncertainty reducing processes explaining HIV risk-related sexual behaviour', *Culture, Health and Sexuality*, 1, 2, 181–191.

Van De Ven, P., Crawford, J., Kippax, S., Knox, S. and Prestage, G. (2000), 'A scale of optimism-scepticism in the context of HIV treatments', *AIDS Care*, 12, 2, 171–176.

Van De Ven, P., Murphy, D., Hull, P., Prestage, G., Batrouney, C. and Kippax, S. (2004), 'Risk management and harm reduction among gay men in Sydney', *Critical Public Health*, 14, 4, 361–376.

Van der Bij, A., Kolader, M., de Vries, H., Prins, M., Coutinho, R. and Dukers, N. (2007), 'Condom use rather than serosorting explains differences in HIV incidence among men who have sex with men', *Journal of Acquired Immune Deficiency Syndromes*, 45, 5, 574–580.

van Loon, J. (2008), *Media technology: critical perspectives*, (Maidenhead: Open University Press).

Waites, M. (2005), 'The fixity of sexual identities in the public sphere: biomedical knowledge, liberalism and the heterosexual/homosexual binary in late modernity', *Sexualities*, 8, 5, 539–569.

Waldby, C. (2000), 'The Visible Human Project: Data into flesh, flesh into data', in Marchessault, J. and Sawchuk, K. (eds), *Wild science: Reading feminism, medicine and the media*, (London: Routledge).

Waldby, C., Kippax, S. and Crawford, J. (1993), 'Cordon sanitaire: "Clean" and "unclean" women in the AIDS discourse of young heterosexual men', in Aggleton, P., Davies, P. and Hart, G. (eds), *AIDS: The second decade*, (London: The Falmer Press).

Waldby, C., Rosengarten, M., Treloar, C. and Fraser, S. (2004), 'Blood and bioidentity: ideas about self, boundaries and risk among blood donors and people living with hepatitis C', *Social Science and Medicine*, 59, 7, 1461–1471.

Ward, M. (2001), 'Making it better: guiding principles for the inclusion of the needs and rights of gay men with HIV in sexual health promotion and primary HIV prevention', London, The Network of Self Help and HIV & AIDS Groups.

Waskul, D. (2003), *Self-games and body-play: Personhood in online chat and cybersex*, (New York: Peter Lang).

Waskul, D. (ed.) (2004), *Net.seXXX: Readings on sex, pornography and the internet*, Peter Lang, New York.

Watney, S. (2000), *Imagine hope: AIDS and gay identity*, (London: Routledge).

Weatherburn, P., Bonell, C., Hickson, F. and Stewart, W. (1999), 'The facilitation of HIV transmission by other sexually transmitted infections during sex between men', London, Sigma Research.

Weatherburn, P., Hickson, F. and Reid, D. (2003), 'Net benefits: gay men's use of the internet and other settings where HIV prevention occurs', London, Sigma Research.

Webster, A. (2007), *Health, technology & society: A sociological critique*, (Houndmills: Palgrave).

Weeks, J. (1998), 'The sexual citizen', *Theory, Culture and Society*, 15, 3–4, 35–52.

Weeks, J. (2007), *The world we have won*, (Abingdon: Routledge).

Wells, M. (2000), 'Sex on the edge', *The Guardian*, London, March 14.

Whittier, D., Kennedy, M., Lawrence, J., Seeley, S. and Beck, V. (2005), 'Embedding health messages into entertainment television: effect on gay men's response to a syphilis outbreak', *Journal of Health Communication*, 10, 251–259.

Whitty, M. and Carr, A. (2006), *Cyberspace romance: the psychology of online relationships*, (Houndmills, Basingstoke: Palgrave Macmillan).

WHO (2006), 'Defining sexual health: Report of a technical consultation on sexual health 28–31 January 2002, Geneva', Geneva, World Health Organisation.

Wienke, C. (2006), 'Sex the natural way: the marketing of Cialis and Levitra', in Rosenfeld, D. and Faircloth, C. (eds), *Medicalised masculinities* (Philadelphia: Temple University Press).

Wilson, E. (2007), 'How to bottle a generation', *New York Times*, Online source, www.nytimes.com, Date accessed: 29 October 2007.

Wolitski, R. (2007), 'The emergence of barebacking among gay and bisexual men in the United States: a public health perspective', in Halkitis, P., Wilton, L. and Drescher, J. (eds), *Barebacking: psychosocial and public health approaches*, (Binghamton: Haworth Medical Press).

Wolitski, R., Valdiserri, R., Denning, P. and Levine, W. (2001), 'Are we headed for a resurgence of the HIV epidemic among men who have sex with men?', *American Journal of Public Health*, 91, 6, 883–888.

Young, R. (2002), 'Sexuality and the Internet', *Science as Culture*, 11, 2, 215–233.

Young, S., Nussman, A. and Monin, B. (2007), 'Potential moral stigma and reactions to sexually transmitted diseases: evidence for a disjunction fallacy', *Personality and Social Psychology Bulletin*, 33, 6, 789–799.

Index

Abstract Sex 16
abundance 30
actor-network theory 24
Adam, A. 17, 41, 64
Adam, B. 94
addiction 6, 19, 27, 52
adherence 136, 158
Adkins, L. 114, 116
advocacy movement 85
   see also HIV treatment advocacy
The Advocate 130
The Age 6
agency of user 70
agnostic position 52
*AIDS: the making of a chronic
   disease* 78
AIDS crisis 132–4
altruism 98, 101, 102, 106, 107,
   108–12, 118, 119–20, 139, 170
   problems for 109–11
   reliance on 109
altruistic individualism 103–4
ambivalence, of gay men 93
anal sex, without condoms 10, 92,
   117, 128, 135–6
anonymity 49, 57, 73, 127, 141,
   168, 169
   critique of 56
   of communication 72
   of internet-based communication
      and sexuality 52, 53–5
   and intimacy 54
   as an organising principle of
      online communication 62,
      64
antibody testing, of HIV 76, 80, 98,
   114, 116
Arvidsson, A. 4, 5, 27, 32, 49, 54,
   59, 68, 165
Attwood, F. 17, 41
authenticity 26, 30, 31, 38, 47, 54,
   72, 122, 125, 127, 166, 168
   and gender 32

authority 124, 166
   decentring of 33, 8, 9
   medical 37–8, 90, 143, 144,
      149–51, 153, 156, 159, 161, 162
   and public health 20, 145–8, 157
autonomy 9, 16, 39, 44, 112, 120,
   139, 140–1, 152
   and gift relationship, tension
      between 102
   sexual 151, 172
avatar, meaning of 25
   see also questing avatars

Ballard, J.G. 17
barebacking 10, 13, 52–3, 93, 94,
   116–17, 140
   and anal sex without condoms
      136
   challenges of 135
   and popular media 132
   and risk-taking 135
   spectacular risk and ethnographic
      interview about 128–9
   and transgression 136
   virtual 132
Bay Area Reporter 130
Beck, U. 23
Beck-Gernsheim, E. 23
Bemygal.com 49
Berridge, V. 106
biological citizenship 42, 44
biological model, of disease 14
bio-medicalisation 36, 48, 126
bio-politics 114, 115
bio-technical embrace 146, 148
bio-technologies 7, 18, 47, 101, 108,
   118, 138, 145, 149–50, 159, 166
   and communication 65–6
   and de-medicalisation 150
   influencing sexual practice 82–3
   and innovation 106–7
   and Viagra cyborg 33, 34
   see also individual entries

Biressi, A.   131
blame   84, 94, 98, 116, 119, 132,
    159, 160, 168
Bordo, S.   3
branding, of internet-mediated social
    relations   4
British HIV Association treatment
    guidelines   82
broadcast media and culture   66–7
Brown, M.   45, 132
Bryant, J.   45
bug chaser   93, 117, 131

Calvin Klein Corporation   3, 4
capitalism   41, 43, 68, 69, 70, 156,
    165
Carr, A.   16
Carter, D.   32, 64
Castells, M.   3, 23
casual anonymous sex   84
caveat emptor   94, 138
Christian dating for free   49
citizenship
    biological   42, 44
    definition of   15
    discourse   39, 40
    and intimacy   43
    somatic   115
    technosexual   15–18, 38–46, 47,
        111, 117, 162, 165, 172
    see also sexual citizenship
civil partnerships   40
civil society   12, 18, 69, 138
CK IN2U   3, 4
Cleminson, R.   17, 18, 24, 120, 165
coercion   41, 105, 112, 115, 140,
    151
Cohen, E.   60
Cohn, S.   153–4
communication   2, 10, 20, 33, 65,
    75, 145
    anonymous   53
    and e-dating   60, 66, 160
    internet-based   54–5, 56, 61, 62,
        64, 67–8, 93, 117, 160
    see also bio-technologies
compliance approach   99, 100,
    155
compulsion   52, 58, 105

condom   50–1, 87, 89, 92–3, 111
    anal sex without   10, 92, 117, 128,
        135–6
    female   7
    negotiation for the need of   90
    and spectacular risk stories   133
Conrad, P.   151
conservatism   43–4, 132, 140, 141
contact tracing   8, 157
contagion   108, 117, 170
    and gift   101–7
Cook, H.   24, 152
cooperation   111, 112, 139, 167
cordon sanitaire   9, 11, 95, 100,
    104
Cossman, B.   40
Cox, P.   105
Crash   17
Crimp, D.   141
crisis discourse   133–4
Crossley, M.   136
Cullen, J.   153–4
cultural pessimism   39, 42–3, 140,
    166
cultural theory, of risk   84
culture industry critique   66–72
cyber-community of intelligibility
    65, 66
cyber-ethics, of reciprocal care   64
cyber-ethnography   16, 31, 52, 67,
    160
    of homosexuality   29
    of intimate online experience   26,
        28, 32, 47, 55, 117, 125, 141,
        166
cyber-feminism   66, 94, 166
cyber-ghetto   57, 58–9, 73
cyber-pornography *see* cyber sex
cybersex   5, 6, 16, 19, 29, 32, 160
Cyberspace Romance   16
cyberstalking   5, 17, 41, 42

decentring, of medical authority   33,
    97, 143, 150, 153, 166
decriminalisation of homosexuality
    40
Deleuzian idea, of temporary
    assemblages   36
Delvecchio-Good, M.   81, 82, 148

de-medicalisation 143, 145, 156
  comparison with
    bio-technologisation 150
  and medicalisation 144, 148–53,
    161, 164
Desperate Housewives 41
differentiated universalism 45
digital closet 49, 56, 73, 130
*The Digital Sublime: Myth, Power and
  Cyberspace* 4
Discipline and Punish 104
disinhibition 53, 54, 55
domestic sex 40
Douglas, M. 84, 115, 135
Dowsett, G. 57, 68, 78

e-dating 4, 5, 8, 40, 52, 125, 129,
    157, 168
  approval for websites 100
  communication and
    bio-technological
    knowledge 65–6
  as cultural anaesthetic 71
  definition of 48
  enterprising individual of 70
  and HIV prevention 64–5
  hypertextual communication 60
  and media 129
  and messaging 60
  narcissistic aspects of 66–72, 156
  overarching rationality of 61
  promoting anti-social forms of
    civic life 69
  and ethnicity 67–8
  readers/writers, role of 60
  as reflexive practice 58–66
  as sexual health risk 49–51
  sites, features of 60
  solipsistic aspects of 62, 66, 68
  and strategies, to avoid stigma
    160
  websites of gay men 92, 99
eharmony.com 49
Elford, J. 51, 82, 93
emotions 27, 28, 29, 61, 64, 84, 90
  and crisis 34
  increase of 148
enterprising individual 70
Epstein, S. 86

erectile dysfunction 149
  medicalisation of 151
  and Viagra cyborg 33, 35, 37, 150
e-stalking *see* cyberstalking
ethics 14, 19, 25, 26, 30, 34, 115,
    125, 131, 133, 141, 166
  of autonomy and constraint 16
  of care 42
  of online social interaction 20
  of reciprocity 29, 31, 60, 64,
    119–20
  and reflexive modernisation 23
  sexual 23, 43, 45, 128
  see also under relationality
ethical relationality *see under*
    relationality
evanescence 23, 30, 32, 60
experiential ethic 32

Facebook 4, 31, 55, 56
falsehood and identity 54, 55
feminism 14, 17, 110, 124, 151
  cyber 66, 94, 166
  and political obligation 46
flaming 53
Flowers, P. 87, 89, 137
forensics 95, 98, 127, 142, 170
  and risk 84, 112–18, 132, 169
Foucault, M. 104
Fox, N. 9, 36, 37, 155
fracturing 88, 137
Frankenstein 34
free choice 70
friendships, in online communities
    32, 42
functionalism 83, 96, 101, 112, 118,
    170, 171
The Futurist 4, 5

gay Disneyland 41
gay men 11–12, 136
  and barebacking 128, 130, 136
  bias towards 10
  e-dating of 57–8, 68, 156, 157
  HIV risk and 82–3, 87, 89, 92–3,
    96, 110, 133, 134, 137–8, 141,
    158–9
  and internet usage 49, 50–1, 55–6
  and post-AIDS concept 78

gay men – *continued*
 and risky sex   94
 and urban sexual spaces   41
Gay.com   49
Gaydar.com   70
gender   17, 27, 43, 44, 66, 110
 and authenticity   32
 and self   31–2
Giddens, A.   23, 26, 43
gift givers   93, 117
gift relationship and
  contagion   101–7
 and blood donation study   102–3,
  106–7
 British approach to sexual health
  care   105
globalisation   24, 71, 165
Gordo-Lopez, A.   17, 18, 24, 120,
 165
Gosine, A.   67, 68, 156
Graydon, M.   117
Greco, M.   14, 15
The Guardian   59, 130

Halperin, D.   10, 128
Haraway, D.   33, 34
Hardey, M.   62, 63, 153
Harrison, L.   55, 56
Health Belief Model (HBM)   83, 95,
 98, 101
healthing-bodies   155
Heaphy, B.   79
Henwood, F.   155, 156
heteronormativity   3, 56, 128,
 136–7, 166
 and domesticity   39, 40–1, 44, 57,
  73, 129, 130
 male   30
 transgression of   136
 and unconscious resistance   136
heterosexual partnering   27, 94
Hijras   105
Hillier, L.   55, 56
HIV bio-technologies and sexual
  practice   75
 effective treatment   77–81
  short-term   79
 hypertechnologisation and sexual
  cultures   91–5

reflexive treatment   85–91
 treatment optimism narrative
  81–5
 see also bio-technologies
HIV Plus   8
HIV prevention   139–40
 and e-dating   64–5
 and individualism   138
 periodisation of   87–8
 rationality of   133
 see also reflexive HIV treatment
'HIV stops with me: prevention
  for positives marketing
  campaign'   109
HIV treatment advocacy   144, 154
 see also advocacy movement
Holmes, D.   67
Holt, M.   138
homogenisation, of sexual culture
 41
homosexuality   10, 40, 55, 56, 105,
 136
 acceptance of   118
 and cyber-ethnography   29
 medical knowledge and the cause
  of   151
Huebner, D.   135
human cyborg   33–4, 37
Huntington's Chorea   42, 138
Hurley, M.   136
hybridisation   33, 38, 95, 166,
 168
hyper-technologisation   47, 75, 76,
 96
 and sexual cultures   20, 91–5
hypertextual communication, of
  e-daters   60

Illich, I.   144
imperative   14, 30, 31, 61, 70, 119
 of psychological individualism
  138
 of public health   12, 19, 39, 94,
  120, 139, 147, 161, 164, 170
 see also individual entries
impermanence   30
 and reproducibility and
  dissemination   60
The Independent   130

individualism 64, 95, 102, 112, 125, 135, 139–40, 167, 168
  altruistic 103–4
  approaches to risk 83–4, 113, 114, 137–8
  neo-liberal 137, 138
  and sexual citizenship 140
informational capitalism 156, 165
innovation
  and imperative 98
    altruism 108–12
    gift relationship and contagion 101–7
    risk and forensic turning 112–18
    technological 4–5, 17, 19, 21, 22–3, 83, 120
    and control of sexually transmitted infections 5
    and Viagra 37
interaction order 63
internet 13, 16
  -based-self prescription 37, 38
  communication 31, 54–5, 56, 61, 62, 64, 66, 67–8, 93, 117, 160
  and health democracy 153–4
  and infidelity 6
  and interventions 2, 7
  -mediated partnering 66
  as a method of surveillance 73
  negative impact of 5, 10
  as panoptic 56, 57
  as screen media 127
  for sexual purposes as drug of choice 51
  as a source of sex partners 50
  see also individual entries
internet-mediated sexual practices 23, 48
  e-dating
    as reflexive practice 58–66
    as sexual health risk 49–51
  narcissism 66–72
  techno-determinism and cyber-perversity 51–8
Internet Relay Chat 60
intimacy 70, 117, 166, 170
  anonymous 54
  and choice 140

and citizenship 43
democracy 27
and popular media 129
reflexive 27
and self 27–8
and sexual practice 15, 17, 26, 66, 122–3, 128, 129, 140–1, 164
of women with online partners 54
IRC (internet relay chat) sex pic scene 29–31

Jordan, T. 33

Keogh, P. 84
knowledgeable, self-regulating patient 147, 153, 155–6, 161
  see also sexual citizenship
Kothis 105

late modernity 26–7, 40, 41, 44, 71, 103, 113, 114, 118, 147, 165, 166, 171
Lather, P. 87, 88
Latour, B. 24
Lavalife.com 49
The Lawnmower Man 22–3, 34
Leiter, V. 151
lesbians 40, 55, 56, 73, 151
liberal democracy 40
Life on the screen: identity in the age of the Internet 16, 28
liquid modernity 23
living after crisis 78
  comparison with post-AIDS 78–9
love bond 27
love of others/love of self 119
Lupton, D. 12, 15, 34, 114, 115

The Mail on Sunday 130
Marcuse, H. 69
Marshall, B. 37
Marshall, J. 31
Match.com 1, 4, 5, 27, 32, 49, 68, 129
matchmaker.com 49
Mauss, M. 101, 102, 107
McGhee, D. 40, 129
McLelland, M. 55

mediatisation
  of narratives of intimate life   129
  of sexual narrative   146
medical authority   90, 144, 149–51,
    156, 159, 161, 162
  decentring of   33, 97, 143, 150,
    153, 166
  reconfiguring, of   37–8
medicalisation and de-medicalisation
    144, 145, 148–53
minimal universalism   166–7
Minitel computer networks   3
Mitra, A.   60
modernity, reflexivity of   27
moral panic   10, 13, 21, 97, 128
  barebacking as   52, 130, 132, 142
  critical geography of   45
Mosco, V.   4
MySpace   4, 31, 55

narcissism   62, 66–72, 73, 156
narrow disease model   11, 12–13, 14,
    123
National Association of People with
    AIDS (NAPWA)   112
negotiated safety   87, 89
neighbourliness   45
neo-liberalism   42, 44, 94, 137,
    138–9, 140
netsex   28, 31, 62
  see also cybersex
Network Society   23
New York Times   3
NHS Direct   7, 155
NHS Online   7
Novas, C.   42, 138
Nuffield Council on Bioethics   98
Nunn, H.   131

obligation, political
  feminist approach to   46
offline   29, 50, 71, 72–3, 127
  meetings   48, 55, 64
  sex   57, 61, 76, 117
  social interaction   54, 56, 61, 63,
    168
online
  barebacking   116, 117
  communication   160

games and interaction   28
  presence   61
  self   54
  sexual harassment   41
  sexual interaction   31
  social interaction   26, 38, 54
  society   31
  see also cyber entries
ontological security   30
  of self   32, 38

Parisi, L.   16, 17
Parker, R.   13, 14, 15
Parsons, T.   101
partnering   26–7
  heterosexual   27
  internet-mediated   4, 20, 27, 48,
    53, 66, 71, 91, 117, 130
  intimate   64
  sexual   42, 48, 51, 53, 69, 72, 112,
    130
partner-protection   95, 104, 110, 111
pastoral power   115
Persson, A.   80, 81
Petersen, A.   12, 15, 112, 114, 147
Phillips, D.   56
Pill, contraceptive   17, 24, 42, 161
  and de-medicalisation   152–3
  and internet pornography   6
  and medicalisation of sexuality
    152
playfulness   55
Plummer, K.   3, 23, 43, 53, 129, 146,
    166
popular media
  and barebacking   132
  exploitation of technosexual
    visibility   130
  and intimacy   129
  see also internet
post-AIDS   78
  comparison with living after crisis
    78–9
post-human anguish   34
post-modernism   44
Potts, A.   25, 33, 36
precarious freedoms   113
prejudice, overcoming   58
prevention altruism   109–10

productive disruption 37, 38, 44, 66, 143, 165
profile uploading, of e-daters 59
promiscuity, virtual 28
Pryce, A. 6, 29, 57, 160
psychoanalysis 53
  and self 28–9
  and transitional space 55–6
public health 143, 170–2
  and authority 145–8
  defining 11–15
  democratic health care 153–6
  dialogical 156–61
  and HIV 39
  and contagion 105
  and imperative of 12, 19
  medicalisation and de-medicalisation 148–53
  and sexuality and technology 6–11
  stewardship model 99
  see also individual entries
public health governance 164
  through danger/cure 167–70
  epistemological strategy for 169
  and HIV treatment 79
  mythical 92
  and relational ethics 38–9
  see also technological visibilities
Purdy, L. 14, 151

questing avatars 25–32, 38, 165–6
quotidian materiality 17, 166

Race, K. 79, 93, 160
radicalism 36, 43, 106, 140, 149
  and democratic culture 85–6
  pessimism in the form of 44
real crime media 131
Reality TV: Realism and revelation 131
reciprocity 30, 31, 38, 60, 111, 168
  ethics of 23, 26, 29, 30, 31, 60
  and giving 101, 102
reconciliation, of reflexive self
  and public health 39
Reddy, G. 105

reflexive HIV treatment 85–91
  engagement with bio-technological complexity 91
  and expertise 89–90
  periodisation of HIV prevention and bio-technology 87–8
  radical and democratic culture 85–6
  re-medicalisation and activism 86–7
  see also HIV prevention
reflexivity 15, 29, 33, 44, 90, 164, 165
  and e-dating 57, 58–66
  of HIV treatment 85–91
  internet-mediated 38
  and intimacy 27, 30
  of modernism 19, 23, 26, 62, 140
  of self 38, 39, 114
reinfection 77, 90
relationality 16, 45, 88
  of ethics 47, 49, 111
  feminist notions 46
  and public health governance 38–9
  technosexual citizenship as 38–46
re-medicalisation 144, 161, 162
  and HIV activism 86–7
  homosexuality 151
repressive desublimation 69
Richardson, D. 40
Riggs, D. 136–7
rights and responsibilities discourse 41–2
risk and forensic turning 112–18
  risk society 113–14
risk individualism 83–4
risk society 113–14, 147, 148, 149
  as Eurocentric 114
risky sex 36, 45, 55, 83, 84, 116, 134, 136
  and barebacking 52
  and e-dating 51
  and heterosexuals 94
  and individualism 137
  sexual partners for 131
Rofes, E. 78
Rolling Stone 130

Rose, N.   14, 15, 42, 114, 115, 138, 163
Rosengarten, M.   138, 154
Rosenstock, I.   83
RSVP.com.au   49, 62

safe sex   45, 77, 82, 87, 88, 109–11, 133, 135, 140, 141
    feminisation of the work of   110
    HBM-related model for   83
    and individualistic action   137
    rejecting   135
Safe Sex Passport   8, 9, 91, 163–4
Second Life   25
self
    autonomous   39, 140
    and gender   31–2
    and intimacy   27–8
    online   54
    ontological security of   32, 38
    portrayed in online communication   62
    psychoanalysis of   28–9
    reflexive   38, 39, 114
    and society   170–1
    sovereign   39, 170
    surveillance of   147
    see also individual entries
self identity   31, 55
self-animation   164–7
self-awareness   19, 20, 25, 26, 27, 32, 54, 87, 168, 169
self-determination   8, 37, 45, 118, 138, 152, 153, 155, 171
self-knowledge   27
    quest for, through sexual relating   28
self-presentation   159–60
self-protection   110, 111, 119
sero-inequality   110
serosorting   89, 137, 138
    internet-mediated   75, 91, 92, 94–5, 97, 100, 113–14
serostatus   57, 58, 88, 92–3, 108, 110, 160
Sex in the City   41

sexual citizenship   13, 14, 15–16, 57, 71, 105, 107, 117, 151, 167
    and individualism   140
    and law   40
    and popular media   129
    and technologies   22
        questing avatars   25–32
        and relational ethics   38–46
        Viagra cyborgs   32–8
    and technosexual visibility   129
sexual embodiment   25, 36–8, 39, 143, 150, 160
sexual ethics   43, 45, 128
sexual health   11, 12–13
    comparison with public health   13
sexual identity   17, 18, 23, 40, 50, 57
    categorisation of   106
sexual instinct   23, 69
sexual liberalism, modern   40
sexual pleasure   13, 171
    and dialogue   45
    and Pill   152–3
sexual practice   169
    of gay men   128
    internet-mediated   23, 48
    and intimacy   15, 17, 26, 66, 122–3, 128, 129, 140–1, 164
    see also HIV bio-technologies and sexual practice
sexualisation of popular culture   41
sexuopharmacy   17, 25, 36, 37, 38, 75
Shelley, M.   34
Slater, D.   29, 30, 102
Smaill, B.   61, 62, 70
social action   2, 12, 19, 39, 77, 96, 98, 112, 144
    and e-dating   61
social context, technological changes into   24
social difference   39, 41, 46, 68, 116, 120
social exclusion, through individualisation   113
social justice   14, 34, 43, 99, 149, 151, 161, 169
    and altruism   112
    model   11, 12–13, 14–15, 57

social obligation   119, 137, 139, 140, 170
  and sovereign self   39, 170
society and technology, relations between   23–4
somatic citizenship   115
sovereign self   46
  and social obligation   39, 170
spectacular risk   21, 125, 142, 164
  and ethnographic media and forensic research   128–34
  and politics of transgression   136, 137
Springer, C.   17
Squire, C.   44
Stephenson, N.   138
stewardship model, for public health government   99, 100, 105
strategic essentialism   43
strategic positioning   89, 91, 92–3
strategic visibility   52, 58, 63, 73, 96
Suarez, T.   136
surveillance medicine   146–7, 148, 149
  and self surveillance   147
Sydney Morning Herald   3
systematisation, of sexual relations   92

technological determinism   11, 19, 82, 167, 168
technological visibilities   122
  medical gaze and Foucault   123–4
  politics of technosexual transgressions   134–41
  psychological knowledge, and individualism   138–9
  psycho-pathologisation, of the sexual practices of gay men   128
  and public health   123
  public/private quality of   129
  spectacular risk
    and ethnographic media and forensic research   128–34
Visible Human Project (VHP)   125–6

Techno-sexual Landscapes   17
technosexuality   2–6, 22
  and citizenship   15–18, 38–46, 47, 111, 117, 162, 165, 172
  dystopian aspects of   5
  governance of   13, 38–9
  social theory of   19
  see also individual entries
thin universalism   45
tiny sex   19, 28
Titmuss, R.   101, 102, 106, 107
Tomlinson, J.   70, 71
transgressive risk-taking   130
transitional cyberspace   55
transparency   3, 20, 64, 65, 72, 122, 125, 127, 168
treatment optimism   81–5, 89
  and knowledgeability   82
  risk individualism in   83–4
  use of forced choice surveys for   82
treatment prescription adherence   158
Treichler, P.   85, 86
triple A engine   53
trust and security   63, 113, 146, 147
Turkle, S.   16, 28, 61, 62, 63

US Centres for Disease Control   108

Valentine, K.   107
Vancouver World AIDS Conference   77
Viagra cyborg   6, 9, 25, 32–8, 75, 143, 149
  biomedicalising effects of   36
  as circuit of technological innovation and medicalisation   37
  and erectile dysfunction   35
  as sexual health concern   36
Viagra.com   1, 37
viral load blood test   79–81
  as technological mediations of self-care and clinical expertise   81

virtuality   28–9, 126
   and barebacking   132
   and promiscuity   28
   of sex and real sex, discrepancy
      between   55
   of sexual space   22
Visible Human Project (VHP)   125–6

Waites, M.   151
Waldby, C.   9, 106, 107, 125, 126
Ward, K.   9, 36, 37, 155
Waskul, D.   16

watershed notions, of HIV epidemic
   77–8
Watney, S.   78
Weatherburn, P.   13, 128
Weeks, J.   23, 40, 43
Whitty, M.   16
Wolitski, R.   135
The World Association for Sexual
   Health   13
World Health Organisation   13

YouTube   56